NEUROSCIENCE RESEARCH PROGRESS

SYNAPTIC PLASTICITY

CELL BIOLOGY, REGULATION AND ROLE IN DISEASE

NEUROSCIENCE RESEARCH PROGRESS

Additional books in this series can be found on Nova's website
under the Series tab.

Additional e-books in this series can be found on Nova's website
under the e-book tab.

NEUROLOGY - LABORATORY AND CLINICAL RESEARCH DEVELOPMENTS

Additional books in this series can be found on Nova's website
under the Series tab.

Additional e-books in this series can be found on Nova's website
under the e-book tab.

NEUROSCIENCE RESEARCH PROGRESS

SYNAPTIC PLASTICITY

CELL BIOLOGY, REGULATION AND ROLE IN DISEASE

GALE N. MCMAHON
AND
RICH G. BUCKNER
EDITORS

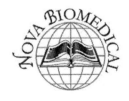

Nova Science Publishers, Inc.
New York

Copyright © 2012 by Nova Science Publishers, Inc.

All rights reserved. No part of this book may be reproduced, stored in a retrieval system or transmitted in any form or by any means: electronic, electrostatic, magnetic, tape, mechanical photocopying, recording or otherwise without the written permission of the Publisher.

For permission to use material from this book please contact us:
Telephone 631-231-7269; Fax 631-231-8175
Web Site: http://www.novapublishers.com

NOTICE TO THE READER

The Publisher has taken reasonable care in the preparation of this book, but makes no expressed or implied warranty of any kind and assumes no responsibility for any errors or omissions. No liability is assumed for incidental or consequential damages in connection with or arising out of information contained in this book. The Publisher shall not be liable for any special, consequential, or exemplary damages resulting, in whole or in part, from the readers' use of, or reliance upon, this material. Any parts of this book based on government reports are so indicated and copyright is claimed for those parts to the extent applicable to compilations of such works.

Independent verification should be sought for any data, advice or recommendations contained in this book. In addition, no responsibility is assumed by the publisher for any injury and/or damage to persons or property arising from any methods, products, instructions, ideas or otherwise contained in this publication.

This publication is designed to provide accurate and authoritative information with regard to the subject matter covered herein. It is sold with the clear understanding that the Publisher is not engaged in rendering legal or any other professional services. If legal or any other expert assistance is required, the services of a competent person should be sought. FROM A DECLARATION OF PARTICIPANTS JOINTLY ADOPTED BY A COMMITTEE OF THE AMERICAN BAR ASSOCIATION AND A COMMITTEE OF PUBLISHERS.

Additional color graphics may be available in the e-book version of this book.

LIBRARY OF CONGRESS CATALOGING-IN-PUBLICATION DATA

Library of Congress Control Number: 2012931079

ISBN: 978-1-62081-004-0

Published by Nova Science Publishers, Inc. † New York

CONTENTS

Preface vii

Chapter I Homeostatic Synaptic Plasticity: Molecular Mechanisms and Implications in Neurological Disorders 1
James P. Gilbert, Guan Wang, and Heng-Ye Man

Chapter II Alternate Calcium-Mediated Signaling Pathways Initiate and Limit Glutamatergic Plasticity Underlying Benzodiazepine-Withdrawal Anxiety 43
Elizabeth I. Tietz and Damien E. Earl

Chapter III Neuronal Calcium Sensor-1 and Synaptic Plasticity: Role in Neurological and Neuropsychiatric Disorders 75
David Fleischmann and Jamie L. Weiss

Chapter IV Faulty Plasticity: A Common Thread Connecting Neurological Diseases 101
Daniel Montoya, Ashley Bofill, and Stephen Gill

Chapter V Synaptic Plasticity in Addiction 125
Yan Dong and R. Suzanne Zukin

Chapter VI	Involvement of Zinc via Crosstalk with Calcium in Synaptic Plasticity and Neurodegeneration in the Hippocampus *Atsushi Takeda*	**149**
Index		**177**

PREFACE

Synaptic plasticity is the ability of the connection, or synapse, between two neurons to change in strength in response to either use or disuse of transmission over synaptic pathways. In this book, the authors present current research in the study of the cell biology, regulation and role in disease of synaptic plasticity. Topics include the involvement of zinc via crosstalk with calcium in synaptic plasticity and neurodegeneration in the hippocampus; convergent mechanisms of drug-induced and activity-dependent plasticity; neuronal calcium sensor-1 and its role in synaptic plasticity and neurological disease; Long Term Potentiation (LTP) and Long Term Depresstion (LTD) in neurological disorders; and synaptic plasticity in addiction.

Chapter I - Homeostatic regulation is a negative feedback response that is similar to other processes in the body that regulate things such as body temperature, hydration levels, pH and osmolarity of fluids, or respiration rates. Each homeostatic mechanism returns the system to an intrinsic physiological "set point". The brain is a dynamic organ that constantly evolves as we perceive and adapt to the world around us. This plasticity allows the brain to learn and form new memories, refine movements, recover after injuries, and to predict and obtain rewards. With billions of neurons making up to 100,000 synaptic connections each, the mammalian brain is a very complex system constantly undergoing modifications as it responds to these changes in the environment. A fundamental question is how the nervous system can constantly undergo modifications without losing its stability or the content encoded within neural circuits. To maintain stability in brain function, neurons must adopt a mechanism of homeostatic regulation by which they can assess the activity levels and make constant adjustment so as to maintain their activity within a normal physiological range.

Chapter II - Prolonged use of benzodiazepine anxiolytics increases the likelihood of physical dependence observable as withdrawal symptoms, including anxiety. Analogous to mechanisms of synaptic plasticity underlying electrical stimulus-induced long-term potentiation, we previously identified increased synaptic insertion and subsequent calcium-calmodulin kinase Type II (CaMKII)-mediated phosphorylation of GluA1 homomeric α-amino-3-hydroxy-5-methyl-4-isoxazolepropionic acid receptors (AMPARs) as a fundamental mechanism underlying behavioral expression of anxiety. On the contrary, drug-induced sources of elevated intracellular Ca^{2+}, which may initiate AMPAR potentiation, and the mechanisms by which CaMKII is activated and deactivated may be different from those central to activity-dependent plasticity. Since L-type voltage-gated calcium channel (L-VGCC) current density doubles upon benzodiazepine withdrawal, Ca^{2+} entry through L-VGCCs, rather than N- methyl-D-aspartate receptors (NMDAR), and possibly through GluA1 homomeric AMPARs themselves may be responsible for the progressive enhancement of AMPAR function after drug removal. While Ca^{2+} influx through NMDARs is not likely involved in initiating benzodiazepine withdrawal-anxiety, a compensatory down-regulation of GluN1/GluN2B receptors, perhaps coupled with the concomitant removal of bound CaMKII limits withdrawal-anxiety expression, unlike following withdrawal from other less selective CNS depressants, such as barbiturates and ethanol. While mechanisms of GluA1 homomeric AMPAR potentiation may be highly conserved, the homeostatic regulation of CA1 neuron hyperexcitability via calcium signaling pathways differs among selective and non-selective CNS depressants associated with the severity of withdrawal symptoms and degree of physical dependence.

Chapter III - Calcium (Ca^{2+}) signaling is the main process that neurons use to undergo synaptic transmission and is a vital mechanism underlying neural plasticity. Neuronal Ca^{2+} Sensor-1 (NCS-1), also known as Frequenin, is an EF-hand high-affinity Ca^{2+}-sensing protein that is an important signaling regulator of neurotransmission. Synaptic plasticity is the ability of neuronal connections (synapses) to adapt both chemically and physically to physiologically relevant stimuli such as the synaptic changes that are essential to learning and memory (e.g. neurotransmission and synaptic maintenance). When this process of synaptic plasticity is distorted, the consequences can lead to both neurological diseases and neuropsychiatric disorders. NCS-1 is involved in both short- and long- term synaptic plasticity. It is located on axon terminals as well as dendrites, and is a regulator of neuronal outgrowth. NCS-1 has also been shown to interact with or regulate neuronal mediators of synaptic transmission. These include voltage-gated Ca^{2+} channels, TRPC5 channels, D2 dopamine receptors, IP3 receptors, and signaling proteins implicated in Alzheimer's disease, Parkinson's disease, and X-linked mental retardation. NCS-1 is implicated in autism, schizophrenia, bipolar disorder, and neurodegenerative disorders. In this review, we give a detailed summary of the current knowledge of NCS-1's role in synaptic plasticity, and speculate about the mechanisms linking NCS-1 signaling to neurological disease.

Chapter IV - Plastic processes, in particular Long Term Potentiation (LTP) and Long Term Depression (LTD), seem to play a role in the development of certain neurological disorders. Both physiological processes are defined by long lasting changes in synaptic transmission and are commonly studied in the hippocampus, although there is evidence of their occurrence in some other brain areas, particularly cortico-striatal networks. It is well known that plasticity is affected in Alzheimer's disease due to a deficiency in N-Methyl-D-Asparte (NMDA) receptors, one of the central elements on which the induction of LTP hinges. The present chapter focuses, however, on recent developments in animal and human studies that associate LTP to other conditions such as Huntington's, Parkinson's, and dystonia. In most cases, plasticity, as indexed by LTP or LTD manipulations, is impaired. In some instances, NMDA receptors are involved together with other neurotransmitters systems. We point out that a unified view of the role of plasticity in disease has not been developed. However, recent models of homeostatic plasticity (a negative feedback mechanism, present in neural populations, that offset excessive excitation or inhibition by adjusting the limits of synaptic strength) may be useful to understand and predict some of the observed effects. We argue that future research has to establish plasticity's contribution, either as a promoter of a given disorder or as a side-effect resulting from other physiological processes.

Chapter V - Drug addiction, defined as compulsive drug use despite serious negative consequences, has been one of the major social problems facing modern societies. A growing body of evidence suggests that drug exposure induces a series of adaptive changes within the brain reward circuitry, some of which are extremely long-lasting and which may mediate maladaptive emotion/reward learning and memory, thus leading to addiction. Here, we review recent findings concerning drug-induced neuronal plasticity occurring at excitatory synapses in the brain areas that make up the reward circuitry. Given that the synapse Drug addiction, defined as compulsive drug use despite serious negative consequences, has been one of the major social problems facing modern societies. A growing body of evidence suggests that drug exposure induces a series of adaptive changes within the brain reward circuitry, some of which are extremely long-lasting and which may mediate maladaptive emotion/reward learning and memory, thus leading to addiction. Here, we review recent findings concerning drug-induced neuronal plasticity occurring at excitatory synapses in the brain areas that make up the reward circuitry. Given that the synapse.

Chapter VI - Zinc is released with glutamate from neuron terminals in the hippocampus. Zinc may serve as a negative-feedback factor of presynaptic activity and negatively modulate postsynaptic calcium mobilization. On the other hand, the hippocampus is vulnerable to glutamate excitotoxicity, a final common pathway for numerous pathological processes such as Alzheimer's disease and amyotrophic lateral sclerosis, in addition to stroke/ischemia, temporal lobe epilepsy. The excitotoxicity is linked to the excessive influx of zinc and calcium. The crosstalk between zinc and calcium via calcium channels may play a role in both synaptic plasticity and excitotoxicity. This paper summarizes the involvement of zinc in functional and toxic aspects in the hippocampus focused on the crosstalk. The enhanced excitotoxicity in the hippocampus in zinc deficiency is also summarized.

In: Synaptic Plasticity
Editors: G. N. McMahon et al.
ISBN: 978-1-62081-004-0
© 2012 Nova Science Publishers, Inc.

Chapter I

HOMEOSTATIC SYNAPTIC PLASTICITY: MOLECULAR MECHANISMS AND IMPLICATIONS IN NEUROLOGICAL DISORDERS

James P. Gilbert, Guan Wang and Heng-Ye Man[*]
Department of Biology, Boston University, US

INTRODUCTION

Homeostatic regulation is a negative feedback response that is similar to other processes in the body that regulate things such as body temperature, hydration levels, pH and osmolarity of fluids, or respiration rates. Each homeostatic mechanism returns the system to an intrinsic physiological "set point". The brain is a dynamic organ that constantly evolves as we perceive and adapt to the world around us. This plasticity allows the brain to learn and form new memories, refine movements, recover after injuries, and to predict and obtain rewards. With billions of neurons making up to 100,000 synaptic connections each, the mammalian brain is a very complex system constantly undergoing modifications as it responds to these changes in the environment. A fundamental question is how the nervous system can constantly undergo modifications without losing its stability or the content encoded within neural

---

[*] Correspondence should be addressed to Heng-Ye Man, Department of Biology, Boston University, 5 Cummington St, Boston MA 02215. E-mail: hman@bu.edu.

circuits. To maintain stability in brain function, neurons must adopt a mechanism of homeostatic regulation by which they can assess the activity levels and make constant adjustment so as to maintain their activity within a normal physiological range (Burrone *et al.*, 2002; Davis and Bezprozvanny, 2001; Turrigiano *et al.*, 1998; Turrigiano and Nelson, 2004).

At the neuronal level, homeostatic plasticity aims to maintain a stable rate in firing action potentials. This can be achieved through adjustments in the strength of synaptic inputs, neuronal excitability, neuronal connectivity or the balance between excitation and inhibition. Among these possibilities, the regulation of synaptic strength has been the most extensively studied and believed the most crucial measure in homeostatic regulation, which is known as homeostatic synaptic plasticity, or synaptic scaling (Burrone *et al.*, 2002; Davis and Bezprozvanny, 2001; Turrigiano *et al.*, 1998).

BASIC PARADIGMS IN HOMEOSTATIC SYNAPTIC PLASTICITY

Homeostatic synaptic plasticity has mostly been studied in cultured cortical and hippocampal neurons (Turrigiano *et al.*, 1998; Burrone and Murthy, 2002; Wierenga *et al.*, 2006). A typical paradigm for studying this phenomenon is to manipulate the global activity levels with a bath application of pharmacological reagents to suppress or enhance neuronal activity. The homeostatic responses are measured electrophysiologically by analyzing the miniature excitatory, or inhibitory, postsynaptic currents (mEPSCs or mIPSCs, respectively). In doing so, one can observe changes in the amplitude or frequency of these postsynaptic potentials after chronic drug treatments. A change in amplitude will reflect alterations in postsynaptic neurotransmitter receptor number, while a change in frequency indicates a presynaptic change in the probability of neurotransmitter release or number of synaptic connections. Following 1-2 days of incubation with tetrodotoxin (TTX) in cultured neurons, a sodium channel blocker that inhibits action potentials and silences network activity, a compensatory increase in mEPSC amplitudes is observed. This indicates that the inhibited neuron tries to recover its activity by enhancing synaptic efficacy (Turrigiano *et al.*, 1998; Malinow and Malenka, 2002; Frank *et al.*, 2006). Conversely, chronic bath application of bicuculline, an antagonist of the inhibitory gamma-aminobutyric acid A (GABA$_A$) receptor that triggers neuronal hyperactivity during the ealier phase of treatment, leading to a homeostatic reduction in mEPSC amplitude, indicating an activation-dependent homeostatic down-regulation in synaptic strength (Turrigiano et al., 1998; Malenka, 2003). These pharmacological treatments do not alter mEPSC frequencies, indicating a postsynaptic-dependent mechanism in the expression of homeostatic synaptic regulation.

HOMEOSTATIC SYNAPTIC PLASTICITY VERSUS HEBBIAN PLASTICITY

Hebbian synaptic plasticity, including long-term potentiation (LTP) and long-term depression (LTD), is believed to be the cellular substrate for learning and memory. Hebbian plasticity is positive-feedback in nature, and over time, an LTP- or LTD-dominant neuron could potentially reach functional saturation or complete silence, respectively. It is therefore necessary for neurons to have an intrinsic sensor of their own activity and the ability to restore its activity to a basal set point. Unlike Hebbian plasticity that occurs at single synapses, homeostatic synaptic plasticity is believed to regulate the entire synapse population of a neuron. Because global homeostatic regulation is believed to scale the activity of synapses up or down proportionally with a fixed multiplicative factor, it is also known as synaptic scaling (Figure 1).

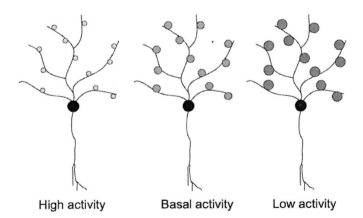

Figure 1. Homeostatic synaptic scaling. In a neuron, when activity is chronically suppressed, AMPA receptor accumulation at all synapses is increased (up scaling, right), whereas when activity is enhanced, receptor amounts are reduced at the synapses (down scaling, left). Red circles on the dendrites represent AMPAR clusters.

However, recent studies demonstrate that homeostatic regulation also occurs locally at dendrites, or even at the single synapse level (Hou *et al.*, 2008, 2011; Turrigiano, 2008; Yu and Goda, 2009). A hallmark for Hebbian plasticity is its synapse specificity; a single synapse can be regulated specifically for a long period of time without affecting the neighboring synapses. Although relatively long-term modifications at the LTP or LTD synapses have important implications in learning and memory, the altered activity still needs to eventually be restored to basal levels in order to maintain brain stability. In this case, homeostatic regulation at single synapses is likely to play a key role in counter balancing the Hebbian plasticity. Presumably, a coupling mechanism may exist linking Hebbian and homeostatic plasticity and therefore, after a certain time, LTP activates the homeostatic mechanism to restore the synaptic activity.

EXPRESSION OF HOMEOSTATIC SYNAPTIC PLASTICITY

Homeostatic synaptic plasticity can be expressed either presynaptically, or postsynaptically, or both. Presynaptic release has been studied by an optical approach using an ampiphillic dye such as FM1-43. This dye has a hydrophobic tail and a positively charged polar head. When cells are treated *in vitro* with FM1-43, the tail of the molecule allows the dye to get into the plasma membrane of a cell (or more importantly a synaptic vesicle during release) and the positively charged head can't get into the lipid bilayer. As more neurotransmitter release occurs, more synaptic vesicles are retrieved back into the presynaptic terminal producing an increase in FM1-43 fluorescence. It has been shown that Ephexin, a guanine nucleotide exchange factor that interacts with ephrin ligands, is sufficient presynaptically for synaptic homeostasis. During synaptic homeostasis, Ephexin functions primarily with Cdc42, a small GTPase of the Rho-submfamily, in a signaling pathway that interacts with the presynaptic CaV2.1 calcium channel. Ephexin binds the Eph receptor (Eph) and it has been shown in Drosphila that Eph mutants disrupt synaptic homeostasis. This suggests that Ephexin/Cdc42 couples synaptic Eph signaling to the modulation of presynaptic CaV2.1 channels during the homeostatic regulation of presynaptic release (Frank *et al.*, 2009).

The primary mechanism in the expression of homeostatic plasticity is to regulate AMPAR synaptic accumulation at postsynaptic sites (Desai *et al.*, 2002; Davis, 2006; Turrigiano, 2008; Rabinowitch and Segev, 2008; Gainey *et al.*, 2009). During homeostatic regulation, AMPAR numbers at synapses are accordingly scaled up- or downwardly in response to activity deprivation or overexcitation, respectively, via alterations in AMPAR trafficking processes such as receptor insertion or internalization (Figure 2). When cultured cortical neurons are incubated with TTX to chronically block sodium channels and silence network activity, the synapse responds in a compensatory manner resulting in an increase in synaptic AMPAR accumulation and the strength of synaptic transmission (Perez-Otano and Ehlers, 2005; Yu and Goda, 2009; Pozo and Goda, 2010). Changes in postsynaptic surface receptor levels can result from a variety of mechanisms working at different levels.

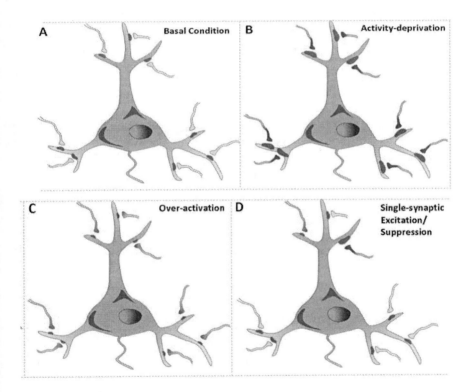

Figure 2. Global versus single homeostatic plasticity. Global activity-deprivation produces a global increase in all synaptic strengths compared to basal conditions (A and B). With global over-activation, a homeostatic response produces downscaling of synapses (C). Homeostatic plasticity can also be seen at single synapses with a selective activation or suppression of activity at a single synapse (D).

Transcriptional, post-translational, intracellular trafficking, or a combination of these have previously been shown to alter receptor surface expression levels. Although subunit synthesis determines receptor availability, and therefore can determine an initial level of control over the numbers and types of receptors present at synapses, several trafficking steps following subunit synthesis appear to operate as regulatory checkpoints for the synaptic incorporation of receptors (Barria and Manilow, 2002; Hou *et al.*, 2008, 2011; Angonno *et al.*, 2011; Peebles *et al.*, 2010; Wu *et al.*, 2011). Activation of glutamate receptors (Beattie *et al.*, 2000; Ehlers, 2000), increasing neural network activity by membrane depolarization, or by unbalancing excitatory and inhibitory inputs to favor excitation (Lin *et al.*, 2000) results in reductions in the synaptic receptor accumulation through receptor internalization, whereas selective activation of synaptic NMDARs can lead to facilitated AMPAR recycling and membrane insertion (Lu *et al.*, 2001; Man *et al.*, 2003; Park *et al.*, 2004). We recently show that continuous activation of a single synapse causes homeostatic reduction of AMPAR surface expression via receptor internalization and degradation (Hou *et al.*, 2011). Therefore, trafficking-dependent alterations in AMPAR synaptic localization serve as a primary mechanism not only for the expression of Hebbian type synaptic plasticity (Malenka, 2003; Malinow and Malenka, 2002; Man *et al.*, 2000; Song and Huganir, 2002), but also for the expression of negative-feedback based homeostatic synaptic regulation (Turrigiano and Nelson, 1998; Wierenga *et al.*, 2005; Sutton *et al.*, 2006; Levi *et al.*, 2008; Hou *et al.*, 2008, 2011; Man, 2011)

A key question in synaptic homeostatic plasticity is to identify the cue molecules or signaling cascades that trigger the recruitment of AMPARs at synapses. Because calcium entry into neurons is intimately related to activity, calcium has been considered as a candidate signaling factor (Turrigiano, 2008; Desai *et al.*, 2009). However, NMDAR-mediated calcium entry, which is critical for Hebbian synaptic plasticity, is not required for homeostatic regulation (Pozo and Goda, 2010; Vitureira *et al.*, 2011), and calcium from voltage-gated calcium channels has been positively linked to this regulation only in a few circumstances (Vitureira *et al.*, 2011). Work from others and our own indicate a crucial role of AMPARs that do not contain the GluA2 subunits, i.e. GluA2-lacking, calcium-permeable AMPARs (Cp-AMPARs). Suppression of neuronal activity induces the generation of Cp-AMPARs. Importantly, the homeostatic response in mEPSCs by TTX-dependent activity deprivation can be abolished when the GluR2-lacking AMPARs are specifically blocked (Sutton *et al.*, 2006; Hou *et al.*, 2008, Aoto *et al.*, 2008).

Interestingly, blocking of Cp-AMPARs after TTX treatment has no marked effect on the enhanced synaptic activity, indicating that GluA2-lacking AMPARs are required for the induction, but not the expression, of homeostatic synaptic plasticity. Recent studies have identified multiple molecules and pathways that are involved in homeostatic synaptic regulation (See *Molecules and signaling pathways in homeostatic synaptic plasticity*).

LOCAL AND SINGLE SYNAPTIC HOMEOSTATIC PLASTICITY

Homeostatic plasticity has been believed to be executed via global scaling of AMPARs at all synapses in a neuron or the entire network, but recent studies indicate that it can also be expressed locally on individual or a small group of synapses (Hou *et al.*, 2011; Turrigiano, 2008; Yu and Goda, 2009; Goold and Nicholl, 2010) (Figure 2). To visualize locally controlled homeostatic scaling, surface staining and fluorescent imaging techniques are typically utilized. Utilizing microperfusion to locally apply antagonists, Sutton *et al.* (2006) show in dissociated hippocampal neurons that rapid synaptic scaling of AMPAR currents, induced by the suppression of network activity, was regulated by local dendritic protein synthesis in an NMDAR-dependent manner. It is also shown that TTX perfusion onto the soma can increase dendritic GluA2 levels but not when it is applied locally to the dendrites (Ibata *et al.*, 2008). This suggests that different homeostatic mechanisms can differentially regulate AMPARs and that these mechanisms could function within distinct neuronal sub-compartments. Hou *et al.* (2008) first described homeostatic regulation at single synapses. In cultured hippocampal neurons, selective inhibition of the activity of an individual synapse results in a homeostatic increase in postsynaptic AMPAR expression. Recently, using light controlled glutamatergic receptors (Szobota *et al.*, 2007) to precisely stimulate the activity of an individual presynaptic terminal, Hou *et al.* (2011) demonstrates that the level of AMPARs at the excited synapses is selectively down-regulated via receptor internalization and proteasomal degradation. This set of experiments indicates that homeostatic plasticity is utilized by individual synapses to maintain synaptic functional stability.

AMPA RECEPTOR TRAFFICKING IN SYNAPTIC PLASTICITY

Ionotropic glutamatergic AMPA receptors mediate the vast majority of fast excitatory synaptic transmission in the central nervous system. AMPARs are heterotetramers assembled from different combinations of four subunits, GluA1-4, the most common of which are receptors containing GluA1/GluA2 or GluA2/GluA3 (Figure 3). As a result of a unique property acquired by mRNA editing on the GluA2 subunit, AMPARs containing GluA2 subunits are impermeable to calcium. In contrast, NMDARs have high calcium permeability, with calcium influx triggering many downstream signaling pathways critical for the induction of synaptic plasticity, such as LTP and LTD. AMPARs are localized at the postsynaptic domain at a high density, and accumulation is believed to be stabilized and regulated by interactions with cytosolic scaffolding proteins such as GRIP, SAP97, PICK1, Stargazin and PSD-95. These AMPAR-associated proteins usually contain one or more PSD domains through which they interact with the intracellular C-terminus of GluAs to regulate AMPAR synaptic targeting, intracellular trafficking, as well as channel function (Tomita *et al.*, 2001; Song and Huganir, 2002; Kim and Sheng, 2004).

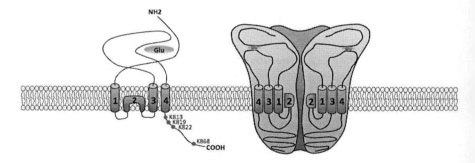

Figure 3. AMPA receptor subunits and the membrane topology. AMPARs are complexes with a variety of combinations of the GluA1-4 subunits. All subunits share the same membrane topology, with an extracellular N-terminus, an intracellular C-terminus, three transmembrane domains and an intramembrane loop. Four heterosubunits are needed to form one receptor channel, which normally contains at least one GluA2 subunit. The last several amino acids at the end of the C-terminal specifically bind to PDZ domain-containing proteins to regulate receptor trafficking. Four lysine (K) residues can be modified for ubiquitination.

A large number of studies have established that AMPARs are not passively localized at the postsynaptic domain. Rather, they are very dynamic, trafficking constantly between the plasma membrane and intracellular compartments (Bredt and Nicoll, 2003; Malenka 2003; Malinow, 2003; Sheng and Hyoung Lee, 2003; Collingridge *et al.*, 2004). AMPARs, like other membrane proteins, are synthesized in the ER and following further modification in the Golgi, are transported to and fused with the plasma membrane, while preexisting surface AMPARs are removed through receptor endocytosis. At basal conditions, a balance between opposing processes, receptor insertion and internalization, maintains the stable cell-surface level of AMPARs. AMPARs are internalized via the clathrin-coated pit pathway, initiated by an association of the receptor subunit C-terminus with the clathrin adaptor molecule AP2 (Man *et al.*, 2000; Lee *et al.*, 2002). On the other hand, cell-surface insertion of AMPARs is mediated by SNARE protein interactions, a ubiquitous machinery for vesicle-based membrane fusion (Lu et al. 2001). Both receptor endocytosis and insertion seem to occur at the parasynaptic sites (Passafaro et al. 2001; Blanpied et al. 2002), likely due to the dense structure underneath the postsynaptic membrane.

AMPAR trafficking, including both exocytosis and endocytosis, is subject to activity-dependent regulation. The resulting imbalance of the two trafficking pathways causes a net change in the abundance of synaptic AMPARs, which has been demonstrated to be the cellular mechanism underlying synaptic plasticity. AMPAR internalization can be induced by application of glutamate, NMDA or AMPA to activate their respective receptors (Lin *et al.*, 2000; Man *et al.*, 2000), or KCl and bicuculline to enhance global neuronal network activities (Ehlers 2000). In contrast, activation of synaptic NMDARs induces AMPA surface insertion (Lu *et al.*, 2001).

A large body of data support that long-term changes in the efficacy of synaptic transmission including LTP and LTD are expressed via alterations in AMPAR trafficking and thus their synaptic expression. For instance, LTP is abolished by reagents that disrupt membrane fusion (Lledo *et al.*, 1998); an LTP-inducing stimulation paradigm drives GluA1 into spines (Shi et al., 1999). In cultured hippocampal neurons, application of glycine, an NMDA receptor co-agonist to selectively activate synaptic NMDA receptors, results in a long-lasting enhancement in synaptic transmission via SNARE-dependent AMPARs (Lu *et al.*,2001; Park *et al.*, 2004). Consistent with NMDA-induced chemical LTD (Lee *et al.*, 1998), activation of NMDA receptors induces marked AMPA receptor endocytosis (Beattie *et al.*, 2000; Lin *et al.*, 2000). In hippocampal slices, disrupting the dynamin-dependent endocytotic process abolishes LTD, indicating a participation of clathrin-mediated receptor internalization (Man *et al.,* 2000). An increasing amount of data indicates a role of glutamate transporters in the regulation of synaptic plasticity (Nicoll *et al.,* 1998; Malinow and Malenka, 2002; Song and Huganir, 2002; Malenka, 2003; Sheng and Hyoung Lee, 2003).

GLUA2-LACKING, CALCIUM PERMEABLE AMPA RECEPTORS (CP-AMPARS)

Under physiological conditions most AMPARs contain at least one GluA2 subunit and allow only sodium influx to depolarize membrane potentials during synaptic activation. When AMPARs are composed without GluA2 subunits, the receptor channel will permit calcium in addition to sodium, causing an inward rectification in the current-voltage relationship (I-V curve). This property of GluA2 is acquired post-transcriptionally by RNA editing at the Q/R site, where a glutamine (Q) codon is replaced by an arginine (R) codon. Because the editing site is located in the channel pore, the positively charged arginine blocks calcium influx. It has been found that the expression of GluA2-lacking receptors is regulated by development, synaptic activity or pathological challenges such as ischemia or amyotrophic lateral sclerosis (ALS) (Peng *et al.*, 2006). In early postnatal development, cortical pyramidal neurons have higher rectification in AMPAR-mediated synaptic currents, which diminishes in more mature animals, indicating a developmental switch in AMPAR composition and calcium permeability (Kumar *et al.,* 2002). By providing an unconventional source of calcium other than NMDAR or calcium channels, GluA2-lacking AMPARs may play an important role in synaptic plasticity. Indeed, inhibitory interneuron studies demonstrate that the NMDAR-independent LTP and LTD are induced by GluA2-lacking postsynaptic AMPARs (Mahanty and Sah, 1998). Recent work shows that even in the conventional NMDAR-dependent hippocampal LTP, GluA2-lacking AMPARs are first incorporated into the synapse, which will then be replaced with GluA2-containing receptors (Plant *et al.,* 2006). In cerebellar stellate cells which normally contain GluA2-lacking AMPARs, high frequency presynaptic activity induces a calcium-dependent increase in synaptic insertion of GluA2-containing AMPARs (Liu and Cull-Candy, 2000). These findings strongly indicate the presence of a self-regulating mechanism by which calcium, via GluA2-lacking receptors, triggers recruitment of normal calcium impermeable AMPARs to synapses. Recent studies indicate a key role of the Cp-AMPARs in the induction of inactivity-dependent homeostatic synaptic plasticity.

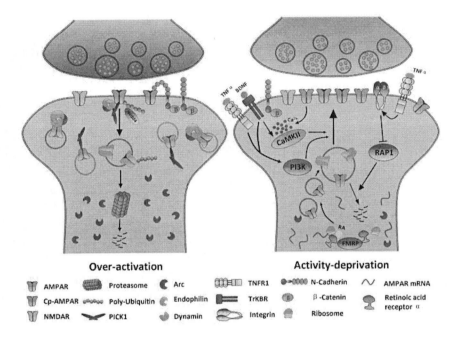

Figure 4. Regulation of homeostatic AMPAR trafficking and turnover. (Left panel) Elevated synaptic activation stimulates the expression of an immediate-early gene product, Arc, which, together with endophilin and dynamin promotes AMPAR internalization. This process also requires the association of AMPARs with PICK1, and Nedd4-mediated receptor ubiquitination and proteasomal degradation. (Right panel) Under activity deprivation, varied signaling cascades are implicated in AMPAR trafficking and synaptic localization. Activation of TNFR1 by glia-derived TNFα, or the PI3K pathway by BDNF/TrKB and TNFR1 signaling, significantly enhances the post-synaptic AMPAR levels. β3 integrin signaling inhibits the activity of RAP1, which is known to enhance AMPAR degradation. Also, calcium flux via the inactivity-induced GluA2-lacking AMPARs (Cp-AMPAR) activates the CaMKII pathway, causing AMPAR phosphorylation and insertion. In addition, retinoic acid receptor α (RARα) and FMRP lead to local synthesis of AMPARs in the postsynaptic domain.

MOLECULES AND SIGNALING PATHWAYS IN HOMEOSTATIC SYNAPTIC PLASTICITY

Although a change in AMPAR expression is believed to be the primary mechanism for the expression of homeostatic plasticity, molecular components and intracellular signaling pathways implicated in this type of plasticity have not been known until recently. New findings suggest the existence of complex regulatory cascades underlying the initiation, expression and regulation of a homeostatic response (Figure 4).

TNFα

Tumor necrosis factor-alpha (TNFα) is an inflammatory cytokine that is involved in inflammation, immune activation, cell death and degradation (Pery et al., 1995; Allan and Rothwell, 2001). In addition to its important functions in immune responses, TNFα is also important in maintaining the neuronal network stability (Stellwagen and Malenka, 2006; Steinmetz and Turrigiano, 2010). TNFα has been found to regulate the homeostatic up-regulation of mEPSC amplitude and post-synaptic AMPARs (Stellwagen and Malenka, 2006). When incubated with medium from TTX-treated neural cell cultures, the amplitude of mEPSCs is markedly increased. Further, the effect on mEPSCs is abolished when exogenous TNFα receptors are supplemented to the medium to scavenge TNFα, indicating a critical role of free TNFα released to the extracellular environment during activity deprivation. To further support TNFα signaling in homeostatic plasticity, TTX-dependent up-scaling in mEPSCs is completely abolished in cultured neurons or brain slices from TNFα knock-out mice. Interestingly, this abolished scaling can be rescued by co-culture of TNFα knock-out neurons with wild-type glial cells. Further, although neurons produce TNFα by themselves, co-culture of wild-type neurons with TNFα knock-out glial cells still abolishes the up-scaling in wild-type neurons (Stellwagen and Malenka, 2006). Thus, TNFα released from glia, but not neurons, plays a crucial role in the induction of homeostatic synaptic regulation. TNFα mediates homeostatic and synaptic scaling not only in cultured neural cell systems, but *in vivo* as well. In the visual cortex of TNFα deficient mice, the homeostatic regulation resulting from activity-deprivation and the ocular dominance plasticity produced by visual deprivation are both found to be impaired (Kaneko et al., 2008).

TNFα seems to mediate TTX-dependent up-scaling by regulating the trafficking and synaptic accumulation of AMPARs. TNFα induces a rapid translocation of AMPARs to the postsynaptic domain in a subunit-specific manner (Beattie *et al.*, 2002; Stellwagen *et al.*, 2005). After acute TNFα treatment, the delivery of AMPARs to the postsynaptic surface is enhanced significantly through downstream activation of the PI3K pathway (Leonoudakis *et al.*, 2008). Its effects on AMPAR trafficking are mainly through TNFR1 but not TNFR2 (He *et al.*, 2011). Of note, the enhanced delivery of the GluA1 subunit occurs faster than GluA2, leading to the generation of GluA2-lacking AMPARs. Calcium influx via these special types of AMPARs is believed to have an important role in the initiation of the homeostatic response (Man, 2011) (see *GluA2-lacking, calcium permeable AMPARs* below). In addition to enhancing AMPAR synaptic delivery, TNFα also decreases the trafficking of GABA$_A$ receptors. Thus, homeostatic regulation of neuronal activity can be achieved via re-balancing excitation and inhibition (Stellwagen *et al.*, 2005).

CaMKs

Calcium (Ca^{2+}) is one of the most important signaling molecules in the nervous system. In neurons, Ca^{2+} transients from ligand- and voltage-gated calcium channels and intracellular calcium stores (Bloodgood and Sabatini, 2007) activate a family of Ser/Thr protein kinases known as Ca^{2+}/calmodulin-dependent protein kinases (CaMKs) (Wayman *et al.*, 2008). Among all CaMKs, CaMKII and CaMKIV are known to be the most closely linked to synaptic transmission and different types of synaptic plasticity (Colbran and Brown, 2004; Wayman *et al.*, 2008), due to their ability to phosphorylate AMPARs to regulate receptor trafficking (Barria et al., 1997; Hayashi et al., 2000). Although the important role of CaMKs in Hebbian type synaptic plasticity has been extensively studied (Malinow and Malenka, 2002; Wayman *et al.*, 2008), their involvement in homeostatic regulation has not been studied until recently. By using TTX local perfusion, Ibata *et al.* (2008) show that somatic activity inhibition induces up-scaling of mEPSC amplitudes and increased expression of AMPARs at the post-synaptic surface (Ibata *et al.*, 2008). This homeostatic response results from a drop in somatic Ca^{2+} levels and reduced CaMKIV activation (Ibata *et al.*, 2008). In another study, Goold and Nicoll (2010) employed optogenetic techniques to excite the somatic area of hippocampal CA1 pyramidal neurons for 24 hours. This lasting activation leads to a depression of both AMPAR- and NMDAR-mediated currents, and a reduction in surface expression of AMPARs and NMDARs. Interestingly, in this study the researchers also identified Ca^{2+} influx and CaMKIV as the mediator of the depression effects. Since CaMKIV is a known gene transcription regulator (Soderling, 1999), both studies investigate the possible role of gene transcription in bi-directional homeostatic regulation. As expected, pharmacological abolishment of gene transcription blocks the homeostatic regulation in either direction, which demonstrates that CaMKIV regulates bi-directional homeostatic regulation via regulating gene transcription (Ibata et al., 2008; Goold and Nicholl, 2010). These studies indicate an important role for CaMKIV in cell-autonomous bi-directional homeostatic regulation. In addition to CaMKIV, other CaMK members may also participate in homeostatic regulation. Knock-down of βCaMKII in hippocampal neurons blocks NBQX-induced homeostatic increases in AMPAR expression while βCaMKII over-expression increases synaptic AMPAR levels (Groth et al., 2011).

BDNF

Brain-derived neurotrophic factor (BDNF) is broadly involved in many physiological processes in the developing or mature nervous system. BDNF is released from neurons in an activity- and calcium-dependent manner (Balkowiec and Katz, 2002). Once released, BDNF binds to the TrKB receptor to trigger a series of down-stream signaling pathways (Carvalho et al., 2008). Given its positive role in neuroprotection, BDNF is considered valuable in the management of several neurological diseases such as Hungtington's disease, epilepsy, and Alzheimer's Disease (Mattson, 2008).

The chronic presence of BDNF enhances synapotogenesis (Carvalho et al., 2008)], and controls synaptic transmission and plasticity at both glutamatergic and GABAergic synapses (Gottmann et al., 2006). In cultured neo-cortical neurons derived from rat visual cortex, BDNF was first found to mediate homeostatic down-regulation of mEPSCs (Rutherford et al., 1998). Application of exogenous BDNF blocks activity deprivation-induced homeostatic up-scaling, whereas BDNF depletion by high-affinity TrKB receptors mimics inactivity-induced homeostatic upregulation in mEPSCs (Rutherford et al., 1998). BDNF is found to affect mEPSCs differentially in pyramidal neurons and interneurons (Rutherford et al., 1998). At synapses formed onto pyramidal neurons, exogenous BDNF attenuates the TTX-induced enhancement in mEPSC amplitudes but at synapses formed onto interneurons, BDNF enhances the quantal amplitude of mEPSCs. Intriguingly, in cultured hippocampal neurons, BDNF treatment enhances mEPSCs in excitatory synapses, likely due to enhanced AMPAR trafficking (Bolton *et al.*, 2000; Copi *et al.*, 2005), which is inconsistent with its role in homeostatic down-regulation. Recently, several studies show that BDNF treatment enhances AMPAR trafficking to glutamatergic synapses, both *in vitro* and *in vivo* (Caldeira *et al.*, 2007a; Nakata and Nakamura, 2007; Li and Wolf, 2011). In cultured hippocampal neurons, Caldeira *et al.* (2007) show that elevated AMPAR trafficking by BDNF is receptor subunit-specific. Surface expression of GluA1 is preferentially increased in the first 30 min of BDNF incubation, leading to formation of calcium-permeable, GluA1 homomeric AMPARs. At a later stage, 30 min of BDNF incubation enhances the delivery of GluA2 and GluA3 subunits (Caldeira *et al.*, 2007a). Enhanced AMPAR synaptic delivery requires the activation of TrKB receptors and the PI3K-Akt pathway (Nakata and Nakamura, 2007), most likely through phosphorylation of the GluA1 C-terminal at S831 (Caldeira *et al.*, 2007a).

PI3K-Akt Pathway

The phosphoinositide 3-kinase (PI3K)-Akt pathway is known for its involvement in AMPAR trafficking, synaptic plasticity and memory consolidation both *in vivo* and *in vitro* (Lin, 2001; Sanna, 2002; Sheng, 2002; Man, 2003; Gobert, 2008). For instance, protein synthesis and AMPAR insertion in late-phase LTP require PI3K pathway activation (Man, 2003; Gobert, 2008). *In vivo*, the PI3K pathway activation is also required for the maintenance of LTP in hippocampal CA1 neurons (Gobert *et al.*, 2008). Consistent with its important role in LTP, PI3K is also implicated in memory consolidation (Lin *et al.*, 2001). However, in contrast to abundant evidence about its role in Hebbian synaptic plasticity, involvement of PI3K signaling in homeostatic synaptic plasticity is not clear. The PI3K cascade is potentially a good mediator in homeostatic regulation. First, the PI3K-Akt pathway is known to induce protein synthesis (Schratt *et al.*, 2004) and AMPAR membrane insertion (Man, 2003; Qin, 2005), processes known to occur in homeostatic AMPAR up-regulation (Sutton, 2006). Second, both TNFα and BDNF, the two major factors that mediate homeostatic regulation, activate the PI3K-Akt pathway and increase AMPAR expression at the post-synaptic surface (Nakata and Nakamura, 2007; Carvalho, 2008; Leonoudakis *et al.*,

2008). Indeed, work by Hou *et al.* (2008) shows a requirement of PI3K activity in homeostatic increases of synaptic AMPARs following activity suppression at single synapses (Hou *et al.,* 2008). Consistent with this finding, a recent study also demonstrates the PI3K-Akt pathway as the mediator of homeostatic regulation. Presenilin can activate the PI3K-Akt pathway by promoting the formation of Akt-activating cadherin/PI3K complexes (Baki, 2004), and the homeostatic up-regulation is impaired in Presenilin 1 (PS1) knock-out mice (Pratt et al. 2011), suggesting a role of the PI3K cascade. Consistently, over-expression of constitutively active Akt rescues impaired synaptic scaling in PS1 knock-out mice neurons without affecting mEPSC amplitudes in wild-type neurons (Pratt *et al.,* 2011). Together these studies clearly indicate the necessity of the PI3K-Akt pathway in homeostatic up-regulation.

N-Cadherin/ β-Catenin and Integrins

Integrins and neuronal (N)-cadherin/β-catenin are cell adhesion molecules (CAMs) that are expressed at synapses and possess important functions in synapse formation, differentiation and maturation, as well as synaptic plasticity (Dalva *et al.*, 2007; Dityatev *et al.*, 2010). Malfunction of CAMs can produce severe problems in the nervous system including abnormal spine morphology, decreased synapse quantity and impaired cognitive function (Chavis and Westbrook, 2001; Togashi *et al.,* 2002; Takeichi and Abe, 2005; Dalva *et al.,* 2007; Williams *et al.,* 2011). N-cadherin is a Ca^{2+}-dependent homophilic adhesion protein that is present at both pre- and post-synaptic membranes (Mysore *et al.*, 2008). It signals through Rho-family GTPases, via catenins, to control dendritic spine morphology and motility (Elia et al., 2006). N-cadherin regulates the surface expression and intracellular trafficking of AMPARs by forming a complex with β-catenin (Nuriya and Huganir, 2006; Pozo and Goda, 2010). The N-terminal domain of N-cadherin also physically interacts with the GluA2 subunit of AMPARs in the extracellular space, promoting spine growth and synaptic transmission (Sagletietti *et al.,* 2007). By targeting AMPARs during endocytosis and exocytosis at the post-synaptic surface, N-cadherin/β-catenin complexes can regulate the bi-directional homeostatic responses of neural activity (Okuda *et al.,* 2007). Over-expression of a dominant-negative mutant of N-cadherin results in reduced quantal AMPAR responses, whereas selective deletion of β-catenin in cultured hippocampal neurons eliminates TTX- and bicuculline-induced homeostatic regulation (Okuda et al., 2007).

Integrins are heterodimeric transmembrane molecules of which many subunits are expressed in the CNS. Previous studies have revealed multiple roles for integrins in synaptogenesis, synaptic transmission and plasticity, as well as memory formation (Chen and Grinnel, 1995; Chavis and Westbrook, 2001). β3-integrin regulates synaptic strength by modulating the surface expression of AMPARs in a subunit-specific manner. Over-expression of β3-integrin in dissociated hippocampal neurons enhances AMPAR surface expression via suppression of RAP1 (Cingolani et al., 2008), a pathway known to negatively control AMPAR trafficking during synaptic plasticity by enhancing endocytosis of GluA2 subunits (Zhu et al., 2002). Since treatment by TNFα increases surface β3-integrin, β3-integrin may be implicated in homeostatic up-regulation of neural activity by regulating AMPAR trafficking. Consistent with this, neural activity deprivation by TTX causes an increase in surface β3-integrin to a level similar to that of TNFα treatment. More directly, genetic deletion of β3-integrin completely eliminates TTX-dependent homeostatic responses in mEPSCs and AMPAR synaptic localization (Cingolani et al., 2008).

GluA2-Lacking, Calcium-Permeable AMPARs (Cp-AMPARs)

Under physiological conditions most AMPARs contain at least one GluA2 subunit and allow only sodium influx to depolarize the membrane potential during synaptic activation. When AMPARs are composed without GluA2 subunits, the receptor channel will permeate calcium in addition to sodium, causing an inward rectification in the current-voltage relationship. This property of GluA2 is acquired posttranscriptionally by RNA editing at the Q/R site at the second intramembrane loop, where a glutamine (Q) codon is replaced by an arginine (R) codon. Because the editing site is located in the channel pore, the positively charged arginine blocks calcium influx. It has been found that the expression of GluA2-lacking receptors is regulated in development, by synaptic activity or pathological challenges such as ischemia or amyotrophic lateral sclerosis (ALS) (Peng et al., 2006). In early postnatal ages, cortical pyramidal neurons have higher rectification in AMPAR-mediated synaptic currents, which diminishes in more mature animals, indicating a developmental switch in AMPAR composition and calcium permeability (Kumar et al., 2002). By providing an unconventional source of calcium other than NMDAR or calcium channels, GluA2-lacking AMPARs may play an important role in synaptic plasticity. Indeed, in the expression of hippocampal LTP, GluA2-lacking AMPARs are first incorporated into the synapse, which will then be replaced with GluA2-containing receptors (Plant et al., 2006). In cerebellar stellate cells which normally contain GluA2-lacking AMPARs, high frequency presynaptic activity induces a calcium-dependent increase in synaptic insertion of GluA2-containing AMPARs (Liu and Cull-Candy, 2000). These findings strongly indicate the presence of a self-regulating mechanism by which Cp-AMPAR-mediated calcium flux triggers recruitment of normal GluA2-containing AMPARs to synapses.

Following the induction of a homeostatic response by activity deprivation, the increase in AMPAR expression is largely dependent on GluA1, not GluA2 (Thiagarajan et al., 2005; Sutton et al., 2006; Aoto et al., 2008), suggesting the formation of GluA2-lacking, calcium-permeable AMPARs. Consistent with this, AMPAR-mediated currents show inward rectification and become sensitive to Cp-AMPAR-selective antagonists philanthotoxin-433 (PhTx) or Naspm (Ju et al., 2004; Thiagarajan et al., 2005; Sutton et al., 2006; Hou et al., 2008; Aoto et al., 2008). Interestingly, multiple signaling molecules that are involved in homeostatic synaptic plasticity including TNFα, retinoic acid, Arc/Arg3.1 and β3-integrin are capable of causing imbalanced GluA1 and GluA2 regulation and Cp-AMPAR expression. The homeostatic factor TNFα is known to cause rapid membrane insertion of GluA2-lacking AMPARs (Ogoshi et al., 2005; Leonoudakis et al., 2008). In retinoic acid-mediated synaptic scaling, the increase in AMPAR surface expression is GluA1 specific, and the homeostatic response in mEPSCs is abolished by suppression of Cp-AMPAR (Aoto et al., 2008). An unbalanced regulation in AMPAR subunits is also observed in Arc/Arg3.1-mediated homeostatic regulation. Knockout of Arc/Arg3.1 results in a typical synaptic scaling of AMPAR-mediated mEPSCs. Interestingly, Arc/Arg3.1 knockout neurons reveal a significant increase in GluA1 surface expression, whereas surface GluA2 shows no change (Sheperd et al., 2006), implicating membrane addition of GluA2-lacking AMPARs. In addition, disruption of β3-integrin induces internalization of GluA2, but not GluA1 subunits, resulting in GluA2-lacking AMPARs at the cell surface. In our own study, we find that homeostatic regulation by single synaptic suppression is abolished by the application of PhTx, indicating the requirement of Cp-AMPAR signaling (Hou et al., 2008). Interestingly, the blockade of homeostatic plasticity is observed only when PhTx is applied during the early stage of activity deprivation (Hou et al., 2008), indicating that

Cp-AMPARs are needed for the initiation, but not maintenance, of homeostatic synaptic regulation.

Arc/Arg3.1

Arc/Arg3.1 is an immediate-early gene product whose abundance at synapses is strictly coupled with neural activity levels. Strong synaptic activation will dramatically enhance the expression of Arc/Arg 3.1 in dendrites and spines while synaptic suppression decreases its expression (Steward and Worley, 2001; Rial Verde *et al.*, 2006). Arc/Arg3.1 is broadly involved in different forms of synaptic plasticity including both Hebbian plasticity and homeostatic regulation (Bramham *et al.*, 2008). Rial Verde *et al.* (2006) find that Arc/Arg 3.1 controls synaptic transmission strength by negatively regulating the surface expression of AMPAR expression at the post-synaptic surface. Over-expression of Arc/Arg3.1 in hippocampal neurons promotes the endocytosis of GluA2/3 containing AMPARs as well as the reduction of AMPAR-mediated synaptic current amplitude. Importantly, knock-down of Arc/Arg3.1 by siRNA abolishes this effect (Bramham *et al.*, 2008). In Arc/Arg3.1 knockout mice, AMPARs show markedly reduced endocytosis and enhanced steady-state surface expression (Chowdhury *et al.*, 2006; Shepherd *et al.*, 2006). Shepherd *et al.* (2006) also find that Arc/Arg3.1 is involved in bi-directional homeostatic regulation of neural activity via regulating AMPAR internalization and endocytosis. In primary neuronal culture, synaptic expression of Arc/Arg3.1 is enhanced after chronic activity deprivation, while over-expression of Arc/Arg3.1 blocks the synaptic up-scaling of mEPSCs and AMPARs induced by chronic activity deprivation. Conversely, in cultured hippocampal neurons from Arc/Arg3.1 knock-out (KO) mice, either up- or down-homeostatic regulation induced by prolonged TTX- or bicuculline treatment is impaired (Shepherd *et al.*, 2006). Activity of Arc/Arg3.1 *in vivo* has also been shown to be correlated with homeostatic scaling induced in mouse visual cortex by monocular visual deprivation (MVD) (Tagawa *et al.*, 2005). In mouse visual cortex, Arc mRNA and protein level in the superficial layers and layer 6 is found to be dramatically manipulated by MVD (Tagawa *et al.*, 2005). Together these studies demonstrate strong evidence about the involvement of Arc/Arg3.1 in the bi-directional homeostatic regulation of neural activity through regulation of the trafficking of AMPARs. It has also been shown that Arc/Arg3.1 directly interacts with endophilin and dynamin to form post-synaptic endosomes which facilitates the endocytosis of AMPARs

(Chowdhury *et al.*, 2006). Using over-expression of Kir 2.1 (an inwardly rectifying potassium channel) in cultured pyramidal neurons, Beique *et al.* (2011) show that Arc is required for homeostatic up-regulation of AMPARs at single synapses (Beique *et al.*, 2011).

Retinoic Acid and FMRP

Retinoic acid (RA), also known as Vitamin A, is best known for its role in regulating nervous system development, including neurogenesis and neuronal differentiation (Maden, 2007; Bonnet *et al.*, 2008). Aoto *et al.* (2008) show that 24 hr TTX+APV treatment, a homeostatic paradigm that induces synaptic up-scaling of mEPSCs and AMPARs (Sutton *et al.*, 2006), significantly enhances the synthesis of RA in both cultured hippocampal neurons and brain slices (Aoto *et al.*, 2008). Application of RA rapidly increases the strength of synaptic transmission mainly through an increase in surface expression of AMPARs (Aoto *et al.*, 2008). Effects of RA are translation-, but not transcription-dependent (Maghsoodi *et al.*, 2008), and are occluded by TTX+APV treatment, indicating an involvement of RA signaling in homeostatic plasticity. In addition, AMPAR regulation is subunit-specific, with a preferential increase in GluA1 compared to GluA2, leading to the production of GluA2-lacking, calcium-permeable AMPARs. A recent study from the same group indicates a role of the fragile-X mental retardation protein (FMRP) in RA-induced GluA1 local translation (Soden and Chen, 2010). FMRP is a dendritic RNA-binding protein encoded by the Fmr1 gene that is involved in the down-regulation of local mRNA translation and protein synthesis (Khandajian, 1999; Mazroui *et al.*, 2002). In Fmr1 knock-out mice, both TTX+APV-induced AMPAR homeostatic up-regulation and RA-induced local AMPAR synthesis are impaired. Over-expression of WT-FMRP, but not mutant FMRP in Fmr1 knockout neurons restores the impaired homeostatic up-scaling of mEPSCs and AMPARs. FMRP is also known for its direct regulation to the translation of homeostasis related protein Arc/Arg 3.1 (Park *et al.*, 2008). Thus, via the effect of FMRP, homeostatic regulation may be implicated in the neurodysfunction in fragile X syndrome.

PICK1

Many proteins, most intracellularly localized, are able to associate with AMPAR subunits. PICK1, a protein kinase C-interacting protein, interacts specifically via its PDZ domain with the C-termini of GluA2 and GluA3 subunits (Xia *et al.*, 1999). Since the same C-terminal domain of GluA2 also binds to another protein GRIP, a competition exists between PICK1 and GRIP in GluA2 binding (Dev *et al.*, 1999; Lu and Ziff, 2005; Steinberg *et al.*, 2006). Interestingly, phosphorylation of the Serine 880 in the GluA2 C-terminus specifically abolishes its binding with GRIP and thus favors association with PICK1 (Lu and Ziff, 2005). PICK1 is also shown to be involved in the AMPAR trafficking and surface expression. In cultured hippocampal neurons overexpression of PICK1 decreases the surface expression of GluA2 in a PDZ domain-dependent manner; whereas disruption of the interaction blocks NMDA-induced AMPAR internalization, indicating that association of PICK1 with AMPAR facilitates GluA2 endocytosis (Terashima *et al.*, 2004; Hanley *et al.*, 2008). Consistent with this, blockade of the binding between GluA2 and PICK1 by intracellular peptide perfusion blocks cerebellar LTD, a process known to be mediated by clathrin-dependent AMPAR internalization (Lee *et. al.*, 2002). More importantly, the overexpression of PICK1 in cultured hippocampal slices not only results in reduced GluA2 surface expression leading to formation of GluA2-lacking AMPARs, but also in the increases AMPAR-mediated mEPSCs (Terashima *et al.*, 2004). In PICK1 knockout mice, NMDA-induced LTD is abolished in hippocampal neurons due to disrupted internalization, recycling and retention of GluA2-containing AMPARs (Steinberg *et al.*, 2006; Volk *et al.*, 2010). By interacting with the GluA2 subunit, PICK1 plays a key role in the plasticity involving the calcium-permeable, GluA2-lacking AMPARs (Gardner *et al.*, 2005) In a specific type of LTP induced by cocaine exposure at the glutamatergic synapses of dopaminergic neurons in the ventral tegmental area, PICK1 directly mediates the switch of GluA2-containing to GluA2-lacking AMPARs (Bellone and Luscher, 2006) Since calcium-permeable AMPARs serve as an important signal in homeostatic scaling (Man, 2011), these findings imply a regulatory role for PICK1 in homeostatic regulation. Indeed, a recent study shows that in cultured cortical neurons of PICK1 knockout mice, TTX-induced mEPSC up-scaling is occluded due to altered AMPAR subunit composition and aberrant trafficking of GluA2-containing AMPARs while bicuculline-induced down-scaling of mEPSC remains intact (Angonno *et al.*, 2011).

Ubiquitin-Proteasome System

The ubiquitin-proteasome system (UPS) is a crucial proteolytic mechanism. The UPS uses a small protein of 76 amino acids, namely ubiquitin, to mark proteins destined for degradation. Following ubiquitination, a poly-ubiquitin chain is attached to the lysine residues of the target protein so that it can be recognized by the degradation machinery proteasome (Hegde, 2004). UPS components are widely distributed in a neuron from the soma to dendrites and synapses (Bingol and Schuman, 2006; Bingol et al., 2010). It regulates many important synaptic functions including synapse development, maturation and synaptic plasticity (DiAntonio et al., 2001). Given the importance of proper protein turnover in cells, UPS dysfunction is implicated in the pathogenesis of many neurodegenerative diseases (Ding and Shen, 2008).

UPS function is closely related toneural activity levels (Ehlers, 2003; Bingol and Schuman, 2006) to control the composition of post-synaptic proteins including PSD-95 (Coledge et al., 2003; Bingol and Schuman, 2004) and AMPAR-associating protein GRIP (Guo and Wang, 2007). AMPARs are directly subjected to ubiquitination, leading to their internalization and degradation (Schwarz et al., 2010; Lin et al., 2011; Lussier et al., 2011). The degradation of NMDARs is also regulated by the UPS (Kato et al., 2005). The involvement of the UPS in homeostatic regulation has been shown in recent studies (Hou et al., 2008; Schwarz et al., 2010; Jakawich et al., 2010). Jakawich et al.(2010) found that proteasome inhibitors cause a slow increase in mEPSC amplitude as well as a slow up-scaling of surface AMPAR expression, which mimics and occludes the TTX-induced homeostatic synaptic response.

Schwarz et al.(2010) found that AMPA receptor inhibition by CNQX, which has also been used as a homeostatic up-scaling paradigm, significantly attenuates AMPA receptor ubiquitination within 30min. In addition to the pharmacological study, expression of a mutant ubiquitin which blocks ubiquitin chain elongation produced similar effects (Jakawich et al., 2010). In our recent study, we utilized light-controlled glutamate receptors to selectively activate individual synapses (Hou et al., 2008). We find that single synaptic activation leads to homeostatic down-regulation of postsynaptic AMPAR abundance as a consequence of AMPAR internalization and degradation (Hou et al., 2008). This activity-dependent homeostatic AMPAR alteration is accompanied by a recruitment of polyubiquitinated protein and AMPAR E3 ligase Nedd4 (Zhang et al., 2009; Schwarx et al., 2010; Lin et al., 2011), and is blocked by proteasome inhibitors (Hou *et al.*, 2011), strongly indicating a key role of the UPS in homeostatic plasticity. Similar enhancement of AMPAR ubiquitination has also been observed in another study in which the researchers found that bicuculline treatment, which was conventionally used as a paradigm for homeostatic down-regulation (Turrigianno *et al.*, 1998) induces rapid enhancement of ubiquitination on GluA2 subunits of AMPARs and results in decreased surface AMPAR expression (Lussier *et al.*, 2011).

HOMEOSTATIC REGULATION IN NEUROLOGICAL DISEASES

In the brain, the maintenance of a stable basal functional state is of fundamental importance for the execution of all the neurophysiology and higher brain functions. Therefore, disruption in homeostatic regulation could underlie altered brain activities and neurological disorders. Long-lasting changes in neuronal activity, including a misbalance of excitation and inhibition, will compromise network integrity and neuronal conditions. Furthermore, since glutamate receptors play a key role in excitotoxicity, abnormal expression of a homeostatic response may lead to calcium overload and neuron death. To date, scientists have only begun to investigate the involvement of the homeostatic response in the pathogenesis of neurological disorders, but a major role is expected to be elucidated in the near future. Homeostatic plasticity is presumably involved in the pathology of Alzheimer's and Parkinson's disease, drug addiction, autism spectrum disorders, seizure and psychiatric problems.

Alzheimer's disease (AD) is typically classified with large levels of neuronal loss as well as impaired synaptic function and loss of memory. A predominant characteristic of AD brains is the presence of amyloid beta (Aβ) peptides, which have recently been studied for their role in synaptic dysfunction. Aβ is a proteolytic cleavage product from the amyloid precursor protein (APP) and it has been suggested that the excess production of soluble small species of amyloid beta can impair synaptic function as well as the mechanisms that regulate synaptic scaling and regulation (Chapman *et al.*, 1999; Fitzjohn *et al.*, 2001; Hsia *et al.*, 1999; Larson *et al.*, 1999; Westerman *et al.* 2002; Li *et al.*, 2009, 2011), and that neuronal activity can modulate the formation and secretion of Aβ in slice preparations from transgenic mice that overexpress APP (Kamenetz et al. 2003). Aβ has also been shown to selectively depress excitatory synaptic transmission onto neurons that overexpress APP, as well as neurons that do not. This depression is dependent upon NMDAR activity and can be reversed with the blockade of neuronal activity (Kamenetz et al. 2003). Synaptic depression from excessive levels of Aβ could contribute to the cognitive defects seen in AD patients and the activity dependent alterations in Aβ production could play a role in negative feedback mechanisms that normally keep neuronal hyperactivity in check. The accumulation of amyloid beta is caused by an imbalance of its production and clearance in the brain. Aβ is eliminated by a range of processes including receptor mediated transport across the blood brain barrier, microglia phagocytosis, or enzymatic degradation. Studies have shown increase levels of the cytokine TNF-α in AD brains (Gong *et al.*, 1998; Orzylowska *et al.*, 1999; Tarkowski et al., 1999). Increased levels of TNF-α are known to cause an upregulation of AMPARs at the postsynaptic surface thereby disregulating the brain's normal homeostatic response. Production of Cp-AMPARs will therefore become upregulated and the increased calcium could also contribute to neurotoxicity and increased neuronal loss. BDNF is found to mediate homeostatic down-regulation of mEPSCs (Rutherford *et al.*, 1998) and recent evidence suggests that decreases levels of BDNF are associated with Alzheimer's disease pathogenesis (Peng *et al.,* 2009; Philips *et al.*, 1991). This could therefore indicate that altered BDNF levels in AD disrupt normal homeostatic regulation leading to diseases progression.

Hyperphosphorylation of the microtubule associated protein tau is another hallmark of AD pathology. This hyperphoshorylated form of tau aggregates into intracellular cytoskeletal filaments called neurofibrillary tangles that can disrupt neuronal synaptic function. One common element that presents with several features of AD is disrupted neuronal calcium signaling. Increased intracellular calcium levels are functionally linked to amyloid plaques, neurofibrillary tangles and synaptic dysfunction (Chakroborty et al. 2011). A recent study shows that homeostatic plasticity is impaired in Presenilin 1 (PS1) knock-out mice (Pratt et al. 2011). Also, over-expression of constitutively active Akt can rescue the impaired synaptic scaling in neurons from PS1 KO mice, indicating an abnormality in homeostatic plasticity in AD (Pratt *et al.,* 2011). It is possible that pathogenic factors shift the threshold of homeostatic regulation so that a normal downturn in neuronal activity triggers an upward over response, which leads to receptor over activation and elevated calcium flux, and ultimately cell death.

Parkinson's disease (PD) is the second most common neurodegenerative brain disorder after Alzheimer's disease (Forman et al. 2005). Aggregated α-synuclein (α-syn) is a characteristic pathological finding in PD, and the aggregation of α-syn into Lewy bodies is a key contributor to the dementia seen in PD. Recent evidence suggests that α-syn oligomers could be the main neurotoxic species, but the physiological mechanisms involved are still not well understood. With the application of large α-syn oligomers to normal healthy neuronal cultures, a selective enhancement of evoked AMPAR, but not NMDAR, mediated synaptic transmission is seen (Hüls et al. 2011). The spontaneous AMPAR-mediated mEPSCs show a decrease in frequency when compared to control neurons, indicating that large α-syn oligomers alter both pre- and post-synaptic mechanisms of AMPAR-mediated synaptic transmission (Hüls et al. 2011). The decreased excitatory synaptic transmission may directly contribute to nerve cell death in Parkinson's disease due to a disruption of the proper homeostatic regulatory mechanisms. For instance, low micromolar glutamate concentrations are found to be toxic in cultured neurons incubated with large α-syn oligomers. The exact function of α-syn at the synapse is still not known, however most studies support a role of α-syn in modulating vesicular presynaptic neurotransmitter release (Murphy et al. 2000; Gureviciene et al. 2007).

Mutations in the PARK2 gene, which encodes the ubiquitin ligase parkin, causes autosomal recessive juvenile parkinsonism (Kitada *et al.*, 1998). Parkin is found throughout the brain, including the hippocampus (Horowitz *et al.*, 1999; Stichel *et al.*, 2000), and experiments in cultured hippocampal brain slices show disrupted excitatory synaptic function after decreasing the levels of parkin (Helton *et al.*, 2008). Parkin associates with PDZ scaffold proteins in the postsynaptic density (Fallon *et al.*, 2002), and parkin ubiquitinates PICK1, an AMPAR-interacting protein that is involved in AMPA receptor trafficking and homeostatic regulation (Joch *et al.*, 2007; Angonnno *et al.*, 2011). These interactions and the observed synaptic deficiencies suggest a disruption of homeostatic synaptic plasticity through the modulation of AMPAR trafficking to the synaptic membrane.

Huntington's disease (HD) is characterized by cognitive, motor, and psychiatric symptoms, including depression, weight loss, and movement irregularity that later develops into severe akinesia, the loss of voluntary movements (Celsi *et al.*, 2009). HD is an autosomal dominant inherited disease and the mutant huntingtin gene was identified to be reponsible for the disease. The huntington protein plays a role in axonal transport, regulation of transcription, exocytosis, bioenergetic metabolism, prevention of apoptosis, and Ca^{2+} homeostasis (Cattaneo *et al.*, 2005).

There is evidence for altered neuronal synaptic protein expression and function in HD. Reductions in neurotransmitters and proteins involved in synaptic transmission, and associated mRNAs, are prevalent in human HD brain even at early stages with little or no cell loss (Cha, 2007). Studies have demonstrated that transcription of BDNF is increased by huntingtion protein and reduced by mutant huntington protein (Zuccato et al., 2001). Interestlingly, reduced BDNF expression is observed in presymptomatic HD mice (Zuccato et al., 2001). Huntington protein has also been shown to enhance BDNF axonal transport via an interaction with huntington-associated protein 1 (HAP1) while the mutant form does not (Gauthier et al., 2004). BDNF is found to mediate homeostatic down-regulation of mEPSCs (Rutherford et al., 1998) and therefore reduced BDNF levels, or alterations in axonal transport, may play a pivotal role in the disruption of homeostatic plasticity in the early stages of HD.

Epilepsy and seizures are due to a change in normal neuronal activity and the result of aberrant neuronal firing. Homeostatic mechanisms are employed to regulate activity within a physiological range, but disruption of these mechanisms allows neural networks to become unstable and cytotoxic. Recently research has suggested that glial cells in the brain do not play a passive role but rather communicate constantly with neurons through gap junctions and can be activated in the brain by various injuries. Alterations in the function of activated astrocytes and microglial cells have been shown in experimental epileptic brain slice models, producing modifications in potassium channels, changes in the glutamine/glutamate cycle, alterations in glutamate receptor expression and transporters, release of neuromodulatory molecules, and the induction of molecules involved in inflammatory processes like cytokines, chemokines, or prostaglandins. (Seifert et al., 2006; Vezzani et al., 2011). Brain injury or the occurrence of seizures can activate microglia and astrocytes to release many pro-inflammatory molecules such as TNF-α, and initiate a disruption in the brain's normal homeostatic response. Pro-inflammatory molecules can alter the neuronal excitability and affect the physiological functions of glia through paracrine or autocrine actions, thereby altering the glial-neuronal communications. In experimental models, these changes contribute to decreasing the threshold to seizures and could possibly induce neuronal death (Riazi et al., 2010; Vezzani et al., 2008). The glial-neuronal interaction through these various signaling molecules can therefore play a major role in modulating homeostatic plasticity mechanisms, disrupting the brain's normal response to altered levels of activity. It has also recently been shown that transgenic mice overexpressing the mature isoform of BDNF show increased levels of anxiety and seizure indicating a disruption of a normal homeostatic response in these disease states (Papaleo *et al.*, 2011).

ACKNOWLEDGMENTS

This work was supported by National Institutes of Health Grant MH 079407 (H.Y.M.).

REFERENCES

Allan S. M. and N. J. Rothwell,"Cytokines and acute neurodegeneration," *Nat Rev Neurosci,* vol. 2, no. 10, pp. 734-744, 2001.
Anggono V., R. L. Clem, and R. L. Huganir,"PICK1 loss of function occludes homeostatic synaptic scaling," *J Neurosci,* vol. 31, no. 6, pp. 2188-2196, 2011.
Aoto J., C. I. Nam, M. M. Poon, et al.,"Synaptic signaling by all-trans retinoic acid in homeostatic synaptic plasticity," *Neuron,* vol. 60, no. 2, pp. 308-320, 2008.
Baki L., J. Shioi, P. Wen, et al.,"PS1 activates PI3K thus inhibiting GSK-3 activity and tau overphosphorylation: effects of FAD mutations," *Embo Journal,* vol. 23, no. 13, pp. 2586-2596, 2004.
Balkowiec A. and D. M. Katz,"Cellular mechanisms regulating activity-dependent release of nativenative brain-derived neurotrophic factor from hippocampal neurons," *J Neurosci,* 22(23), 2002.
Barria A, Malinow R. "Subunit-specific NMDA receptor trafficking to synapses." *Neuron,* vol. 35, 345–353, 2002.
Barria A., D. Muller, V. Derkach, et al.,"Regulatory phosphorylation of AMPA-type glutamate receptors by CaM-KII during long-term potentiation," *Science,* vol. 276, no. 5321, pp. 2042-2045, 1997.
Beattie E. C., Carroll R. C., Yu X., Morishita W., Yasuda H., von Zastrow M. and Malenka R. C. "Regulation of AMPA receptor endocytosis by a signaling mechanism shared with LTD," *Nat Neurosci* 3, 1291-1300, 2000.
Beattie E. C., D. Stellwagen, W. Morishita, et al.,"Control of synaptic strength by glial TNFalpha," *Science,* vol. 295, no. 5563, pp. 2282-2285, 2002.

Beique J. C., Y. Na, D. Kuhl, et al.,"Arc-dependent synapse-specific homeostatic plasticity," *Proc Natl Acad Sci U S A*, vol. 108, no. 2, pp. 816-821, 2011.

Bellone A. and C. Luscher,"Cocaine triggered AMPA receptor redistribution is reversed in vivo by mGluR-dependent long-term depression," *Nature Neuroscience*, vol. 9, no. 5, pp. 636-641, 2006.

Bingol A. and E. M. Schuman,"A proteasome-sensitive connection between PSD-95 and GluR1 endocytosis," *Neuropharmacology*, vol. 47, no. 5, pp. 755-763, 2004.

Bingol A. and E. M. Schuman,"Activity-dependent dynamics and sequestration of proteasomes in dendritic spines," *Nature*, vol. 441, no., pp. 1144-1148, 2006.

Bingol A., C. F. Wang, D. Arnott, et al.,"Autophosphorylated CaMKII alpha Acts as a Scaffold to Recruit Proteasomes to Dendritic Spines," *Cell*, vol. 140, no. 4, pp. 567-578, 2010.

Blanpied T. A., Scott D. B. and Ehlers M. D. Dynamics and regulation of clathrin coats at specialized endocytic zones of dendrites and spines. *Neuron* 36, 435-449, 2002.

Bloodgood B. L. and B. L. Sabatini,"Ca(2+) signaling in dendritic spines," *Curr Opin Neurobiol*, vol. 17, no. 3, pp. 345-351, 2007.

Bolton M. M., A. J. Pittman, and D. C. Lo,"Brain-derived neurotrophic factor differentially regulates excitatory and inhibitory synaptic transmission in hippocampal cultures," *J Neurosci*, vol. 20, no. 9, pp. 3221-3232, 2000.

Bonnet A., K. Touyarot, S. Alfos, et al.,"Retinoic acid restores adult hippocampal neurogenesis and reverses spatial memory deficit in vitamin A deprived rats," *PLoS One*, vol. 3, no. 10, pp. e3487, 2008.

Bramham A. R., P. F. Worley, M. J. Moore, et al.,"The Immediate Early Gene Arc/Arg3.1: Regulation, Mechanisms, and Function," *Journal of Neuroscience*, vol. 28, no. 46, pp. 11760-11767, 2008.

Bredt D. S. and Nicoll R. A. "AMPA receptor trafficking at excitatory synapses," *Neuron* 40, 361-379, 2003.

Burnashev, N., Monyer, H., Seeburg, P.H., and Sakmann, B. "Divalent ion permeability of AMPA receptor channels is dominated by the edited form of a single subunit," *Neuron*.1992; 8, 189–198, 1992.

Burrone J, O'Byrne M, Murthy VN "Multiple forms of synaptic plasticity triggered by selective suppression of activity in individual neurons," *Nature*. 2002; 420:414–418, 2002.

Caldeira M. V., C. V. Melo, D. B. Pereira, et al,"Brain-derived neurotrophic factor regulates the expression and synaptic delivery of alpha-amino-3-

hydroxy-5-methyl-4-isoxazole propionic acid receptor subunits in hippocampal neurons," *J Biol Chem,* vol. 282, no. 17, pp. 12619-12628, 2007.

Carvalho A. L., M. V. Caldeira, S. D. Santos, et al.,"Role of the brain-derived neurotrophic factor at glutamatergic synapses," *Cell.* 2011; 147(3):615-28.

Cattaneo E., C. Zuccato, and M. Tartari. "Normal huntingtin function: an alternative approach to Huntington's disease," *Nat Rev Neurosci,* 6: 919–930, 2005.

Celsi F., P. Pizzo, M. Brini, S. Leo, C. Fotino, P. Pinton, and R. Rizzuto."Mitochondria, calcium and cell death: a deadly triad in neurodegeneration," *Biochim Biophys Acta.,* 1787: 335–344, 2009.

Cha, J.H. "Transcriptional signatures in Huntington's disease," *Prog. Neurobiol.* 83, 228–248, 2007.

Chakroborty S, Stutzmann GE. "Early calcium dysregulation in Alzheimer's disease: setting the stage for synaptic dysfunction," *Sci China Life Sci.,* 54(8):752-62, 2001.

Chapman PF, White GL, Jones MW, Cooper-Blacketer D, Marshall VJ, Irizarry M, Younkin L, Good MA, Bliss TV, Hyman BT, et al. "Impaired synaptic plasticity and learning in aged amyloid precursor protein transgenic mice," *Nat. Neurosci.* 1999, 2, 271–276, 1999.

Chavis P. and G. Westbrook,"Integrins mediate functional pre- and postsynaptic maturation at a hippocampal synapse," *Nature,* vol. 411, no. 6835, pp. 317-321, 2001.

Chen A. M. and A. D. Grinnell,"Integrins and modulation of transmitter release from motor nerve terminals by stretch," *Science,* vol. 269, no. 5230, pp. 1578-1580, 1995.

Chowdhury, J. D. Shepherd, H. Okuno, et al.,"Arc/Arg3.1 interacts with the endocytic machinery to regulate AMPA receptor trafficking," *Neuron,* vol. 52, no. 3, pp. 445-459, 2006.

Cingolani L. A., A. Thalhammer, L. M. Yu, et al.,"Activity-dependent regulation of synaptic AMPA receptor composition and abundance by beta3 integrins," *Neuron,* vol. 58, no. 5, pp. 749-762, 2008.

Colbran R. J. and A. M. Brown,"Calcium/calmodulin-dependent protein kinase II and synaptic plasticity," *Curr Opin Neurobiol,* vol. 14, no. 3, pp. 318-327, 2004.

Colledge M., E. M. Snyder, R. A. Crozier, et al.,"Ubiquitination regulates PSD-95 degradation and AMPA receptor surface expression," *Neuron,* vol. 40, no. 3, pp. 595-607, 2003.

Collingridge G. L., Isaac J. T. and Wang Y. T. "Receptor trafficking and synaptic plasticity," *Nat Rev Neurosci* 5, 952-962, 2004.

Copi A., K. Jungling, and K. Gottmann,"Activity- and BDNF-induced plasticity of miniaturesynaptic currents in ES cell-derived neurons integrated in a neocortical network,"*J Neurophysiol.*, 94(6):4538-43, 2005.

Dalva M. B., A. C. McClelland, and M. S. Kayser,"Cell adhesion molecules: signalling functions at the synapse," *Nature Reviews Neuroscience,* vol. 8, no. 3, pp. 206-220, 2007.

Davis G. W.,"Homeostatic Control of Neural Activity: From Phenomenology to Molecular Design," *Annu Rev Neurosci,* pp. 307-323, 2006.

Desai N. S., R. H. Cudmore, S. B. Nelson, et al.,"Critical periods for experience-dependent synaptic scaling in visual cortex," *Nat Neurosci,* vol. 5, no. 8, pp. 783-789, 2002.

Dev K. K., A. Nishimune, J. M. Henley, et al.,"The protein kinase C alpha binding protein PICK1 interacts with short but not long form alternative splice variants of AMPA receptor subunits," *Neuropharmacology,* vol. 38, no. 5, pp. 635-644, 1999.

DiAntonio A., A. P. Haghighi, S. L. Portman, et al.,"Ubiquitination-dependent mechanisms regulate synaptic growth and function," *Nature,* vol. 412, no. 6845, pp. 449-452, 2001.

Ding M. and K. Shen,"The role of the ubiquitin proteasome system in synapse remodeling and neurodegenerative diseases," *Bioessays,* vol. 30, no. 11-12, pp. 1075-1083, 2008.

Dityatev A., M. Schachner, and P. Sonderegger,"The dual role of the extracellular matrix in synaptic plasticity and homeostasis," *Nat Rev Neurosci.*, (11):735-46, 2010.

Ehlers M. D. "Reinsertion or degradation of AMPA receptors determined by activity-dependent endocytic sorting," *Neuron* 28, 511-525, 2000.

Ehlers M. D.,"Activity level controls postsynaptic composition and signaling via the ubiquitin-proteasome system," *Nat Neurosci,* vol. 6, no. 3, pp. 231-242, 2003.

Elia L. P., M. Yamamoto, K. L. Zang, et al.,p120 "Catenin regulates dendritic spine and synapse development through Rho-family GTPases and cadherins," *Neuron,* vol. 51, no. 1, pp. 43-56, 2006.

Fitzjohn SM, Morton RA, Kuenzi F, Rosahl TW, Shearman M, Lewis H, Smith D, Reynolds DS, Davies CH and Collingridge GL, et al. "Age-related impairment of synaptic transmission but normal long-term potentiation in transgenic mice that over-express the human APP695SWE mutant form of amyloid precursor protein," *J. Neurosci.*,21, 4691–4698, 2001.

Frank CA, Pielage J, Davis GW."A presynaptic homeostatic signaling system composed of the Eph receptor, ephexin, Cdc42, and CaV2.1 calcium channels,"*Neuron.* 2009; 61:556–569, 2009.

Frank, C. A., Kennedy, M. J., Goold, C. P., Marek, K. W., and Davis, G. W. "Mechanisms underlying the rapid induction and sustained expression of synaptic homeostasis," *Neuron,* 52, 663-677, 2006.

Gainey M. A., J. R. Hurvitz-Wolff, M. E. Lambo, et al.,"Synaptic scaling requires the GluR2 subunit of the AMPA receptor," *J Neurosci*, vol. 29, no. 20, pp. 6479-6489, 2009.

Gardner S. M., K. Takamiya, J. Xia, et al.,"Calcium-permeable AMPA receptor plasticity is mediated by subunit-specific interactions with PICK1 and NSF," *Neuron*, vol. 45, no. 6, pp. 903-915, 2005.

Gauthier, L.R. et al. "Huntingtin controls neurotrophic support and survival of neurons by enhancing BDNF vesicular transport along microtubules," *Cell*, 118, 127–138, 2004.

Gobert A., L. Topolnik, M. Azzi, et al.,"Forskolin induction of late-LTP and up-regulation of 5' TOP mRNAs translation via mTOR, ERK, and PI3K in hippocampal pyramidal cells," *J Neurochem*, vol. 106, no. 3, pp. 1160-1174, 2008.

Goold C. P. and R. A. Nicoll,"Single-cell optogenetic excitation drives homeostatic synaptic depression," *Neuron*, vol. 68, no. 3, pp. 512-528, 2010.

Gong C., Qin Z., Betz A. L., Liu X. H. and Yang G.Y. "Cellular localization of tumor necrosis factor alpha following focal cerebral ischemia in mice," *Brain Research,* 801: 1-8, 1998.

Gottmann K., T. Mittmann, and V. Lessmann,"BDNF signaling in the formation, maturation and plasticity of glutamatergic and GABAergic synapses," *Exp Brain Res,* vol. 199, no. 3-4, pp. 203-34, 2009.

Groth R. D. and R. W. Tsien,"A role for retinoic acid in homeostatic plasticity," *Neuron,* vol. 60, no. 2, pp. 192-194, 2008.

Groth R. D., M. Lindskog, T. C. Thiagarajan,L. Li, R. W. Tsien. "Beta Ca2+/CaM-dependent kinase type II triggers upregulation of GluA1 to coordinate adaptation to synaptic inactivity in hippocampal neurons," *Proc Natl Acad Sci* U S A, 108(2):828-33, 2011.

Guo L. and Y. Wang,"Glutamate stimulates glutamate receptor interacting protein 1 degradation by ubiquitin-proteasome system to regulate surface expression of GluR2," *Neuroscience,* vol. 145, no. 1, pp. 100-109, 2007.

Gureviciene I, Gurevicius K, Tanila H. "Role of alpha-synuclein in synaptic glutamate release," *Neurobiol Dis,* 28(1):83-9, 2007.

Hanley J. G.,"PICK1: a multi-talented modulator of AMPA receptor trafficking," *Pharmacol Ther,* vol. 118, no. 1, pp. 152-160, 2008.

Hayashi Y., S. H. Shi, J. A. Esteban, et al.,"Driving AMPA receptors into synapses by LTP and CaMKII: Requirement for GluR1 and PDZ domain interaction," *Science,* vol. 287, no. 5461, pp. 2262-2267, 2000.

He P., Q. Liu, J. Wu, et al.,"Genetic deletion of TNF receptor suppresses excitatory synaptic transmission via reducing AMPA receptor synaptic localization in cortical neurons," *FASEB J,* vol. 26, pp. fj.11-192716, 2011.

Hegde A. N.,"Ubiquitin-proteasome-mediated local protein degradation and synaptic plasticity," *Prog Neurobiol,* vol. 73, no. 5, pp. 311-357, 2004.

Helton T. D.,T. Otsuka, M. C. Lee, Y. Mu, M. D. Ehlers. "Pruning and loss of excitatory synapses by the parkin ubiquitin ligase," *Proc. Nat. Acad. Sci. USA.*2008; 105, 19492–19497, 2008.

Horowitz J. M., J. Myers, M. K. Stachowiak, G. Torres. "Identification and distribution of Parkin in rat brain," *Neuroreport,* 10, 3393–3397, 1999.

Hou Q. M., J. Gilbert, and H. Y. Man,"Homeostatic Regulation of AMPA receptor trafficking and degradation by light-controlled single-synaptic activation," *Neuron,* vol. 72, no.5, pp. 806-818, 2011.

Hou Q., D. Zhang, L. Jarzylo, et al.,"Homeostatic regulation of AMPA receptor expression at single hippocampal synapses," *Proc Natl Acad Sci U S A,* vol. 105, no. 2, pp. 775-780, 2008.

Hsia AY, Masliah E, McConlogue L, Yu GQ, Tatsuno G, Hu K, Kholodenko D, Malenka RC, Nicoll RA and Mucke L. "Plaque-independent disruption of neural circuits in Alzheimer's disease mouse models," *Proc. Natl. Acad. Sci.* USA, 96, 3228–3233, 1999.

Hüls S, Högen T, Vassallo N, Danzer KM, Hengerer B, Giese A, Herms J. "AMPA-receptor-mediated excitatory synaptic transmission is enhanced by iron-induced α-synuclein oligomers," *J Neurochem,*117(5):868-78, 2011.

Ibata K., Q. Sun, and G. G. Turrigiano,"Rapid synaptic scaling induced by changes in postsynaptic firing," *Neuron,* vol. 57, no. 6, pp. 819-826, 2008.

Jakawich S. K., R. M. Neely, S. N. Djakovic, et al.,"An essential postsynaptic role for the ubiquitin proteasome system in slow homeostatic synaptic plasticity in cultured hippocampal neurons," *Neuroscience,* vol. 171, no. 4, pp. 1016-1031, 2010.

Jin M., N. Shepardson, T. Yang, G. Chen, D. Walsh, D. J. Selkoe."Soluble amyloid beta-protein dimers isolated from Alzheimer cortex directly induce Tau hyperphosphorylation and neuritic degeneration, " *Proc Natl Acad Sci U S A,*108(14):5819-24, 2011.

Joch M., A. R.Ase, C. X. Chen, et al.,"Parkin-mediated monoubiquitination of the PDZ protein PICK1 regulates the activity of acid-sensing ion channels," Mol Biol Cell, 18, 3105–3118, 2007.

Ju W., W. Morishita, J. Tsui, et al.,"Activity-dependent regulation of dendritic synthesis and trafficking of AMPA receptors," *Nat Neurosci,* vol. 7, no. 3, pp. 244-253, 2004.

Kamenetz F., T. Tomita, H. Hsieh, G. Seabrook, D. Borchelt, T. Iwatsubo, S. Sisodia, R. Malinow. "APP processing and synaptic function," *Neuron.* 2003; 37(6):925-37, 2003.

Kaneko M., D. Stellwagen, R. C. Malenka, M. P. Stryker. "Tumor necrosis factor-alpha mediates one component of competitive, experience-dependent plasticity in developing visual cortex," *Neuron,*58(5):673-80, 2008.

Kato A., N. Rouach, R. A. Nicoll, et al.,"Activity-dependent NMDA receptor degradation mediated by retrotranslocation and ubiquitination," *Proc Natl Acad Sci U S A,* vol. 102, no. 15, pp. 5600-5605, 2005.

Khandjian A. W.,"Biology of the fragile X mental retardation protein, an RNA-binding protein," *Biochem Cell Biol,* vol. 77, no. 4, pp. 331-342, 1999.

Kim E. and M. Sheng. "PDZ domain proteins of synapses, " *Nat Rev Neurosci* 5, 771-781, 2004.

Kitada T,Asakawa S,Hattori N, Matsumine H, Yamamura Y, Minoshima S, Yokochi M, Mizuno Y, Shimizu N. "Mutations in the parkin gene cause autosomal recessive juvenile parkinsonism, " *Nature,*392, 605–608, 1998.

Kumar S. S., A. Bacci, V. Kharazia, et al.,"A developmental switch of AMPA receptor subunits in neocortical pyramidal neurons," *J Neurosci,* vol. 22, no. 8, pp. 3005-3015., 2002.

Larson J, Lynch G, Games D and Seubert P. "Alterations in synaptic transmission and long-term potentiation in hippocampal slices from young and aged PDAPP mice.," *Brain Res.,* 840, 23–35, 1999.

Lee H. K., Kameyama K., Huganir R. L. and Bear M. F. "NMDA induces long-term synaptic depression and dephosphorylation of the GluR1 subunit of AMPA receptors in hippocampus," *Neuron* 21, 1151-1162, 1998.

Lee S. H., Liu L., Wang Y. T. and Sheng M. "Clathrin adaptor AP2 and NSF interact with overlapping sites of GluR2 and play distinct roles in AMPA receptor trafficking and hippocampal LTD," *Neuron* 36, 661-674, 2002.

Leonoudakis D., P. Zhao, and E. C. Beattie,"Rapid tumor necrosis factor alpha-induced exocytosis of glutamate receptor 2-lacking AMPA receptors to extrasynaptic plasma membrane potentiates excitotoxicity," *J Neurosci,* vol. 28, no. 9, pp. 2119-2130, 2008.

Levi S, Schweizer C, Bannai H, Pascual O, Charrier C, and Triller A. "Homeostatic regulation of synaptic GlyR numbers driven by lateral diffusion," *Neuron.* 2008; 59, 261-273, 2008.

Li S, Hong S, Shepardson NE, Walsh D, Shankar GM, Selkoe D. "Soluble oligomers of amyloid beta protein facilitate hippocampal long-term depression by disrupting neuronal glutamate uptake," *Neuron,* 62:788-801, 2009.

Li X. and M. E. Wolf,"Brain-derived neurotrophic factor rapidly increases AMPA receptor surface expression in rat nucleus accumbens," *Eur J Neurosci,* vol. 34, no. 2, pp. 190-8, 2011.

Lin A. H., S. H. Yeh, K. T. Lu, et al.,"A role for the PI-3 kinase signaling pathway in fear conditioning and synaptic plasticity in the amygdala," *Neuron,* vol. 31, no. 5, pp. 841-851, 2001.

Lin A., Q. Hou, L. Jarzylo, et al.,"Nedd4-mediated AMPA receptor ubiquitination regulates receptor turnover and trafficking," *J Neurochem,* vol. 119, no. 1, 27-39, 2011.

Lin J. W., Ju W., Foster K., Lee S. H., Ahmadian G., Wyszynski M., Wang Y. T. and Sheng M. "Distinct molecular mechanisms and divergent endocytotic pathways of AMPA receptor internalization," *Nat Neurosci* 3, 1282-1290, 2000.

Liu S. Q. and S. G. Cull-Candy,"Synaptic activity at calcium-permeable AMPA receptors induces a switch in receptor subtype," *Nature,* vol. 405, no. 6785, pp. 454-458., 2000.

Lledo P. M., Zhang X., Sudhof T. C., Malenka R. C. and Nicoll R. A. "Postsynaptic membrane fusion and long-term potentiation," *Science* 279, 399-403, 1998.

Lu W. and E. B. Ziff,"PICK1 interacts with ABP/GRIP to regulate AMPA receptor trafficking," *Neuron,* vol. 47, no. 3, pp. 407-421, 2005.

Lu W., Man H., Ju W., Trimble W. S., MacDonald J. F. and Wang Y. T. "Activation of synaptic NMDA receptors induces membrane insertion of new AMPA receptors and LTP in cultured hippocampal neurons," *Neuron* 29, 243-254, 2001.

Lussier M. P., Y. Nasu-Nishimura, and K. W. Roche,"Activity-dependent ubiquitination of the AMPA receptor subunit GluA2," *J Neurosci*, vol. 31, no. 8, pp. 3077-3081, 2011.

Maden,"Retinoic acid in the development, regeneration and maintenance of the nervous system," Nat Rev Neurosci, vol. 8, no. 10, pp. 755-765, 2007.

Maghsoodi, M. M. Poon, C. I. Nam, et al.,"Retinoic acid regulates RARalpha-mediated control of translation in dendritic RNA granules during homeostatic synaptic plasticity," *Proc Natl Acad Sci U S A*, vol. 105, no. 41, pp. 16015-16020, 2008.

Mahanty N. K. and Sah P. "Calcium-permeable AMPA receptors mediate long-term potentiation in interneurons in the amygdala," *Nature* 394, 683-687, 1998.

Malenka R. C. "Synaptic plasticity and AMPA receptor trafficking," *Ann N Y Acad Sci* 1003, 1-11, 2003.

Malinow R. and R. C. Malenka,"AMPA receptor trafficking and synaptic plasticity," *Annu Rev Neurosci*, vol. 25, pp. 103-126, 2002.

Malinow R. "AMPA receptor trafficking and long-term potentiation," *Philos Trans R Soc Lond B Biol Sci* 358, 707-714, 2003.

Man H. Y., Lin J. W., Ju W. H., Ahmadian G., Liu L., Becker L. E., Sheng M. and Wang Y. T. "Regulation of AMPA receptor-mediated synaptic transmission by clathrin-dependent receptor internalization," *Neuron* 25, 649-662, 2000.

Man H. Y., Q. Wang, W. Y. Lu, et al.,"Activation of PI3-kinase is required for AMPA receptor insertion during LTP of mEPSCs in cultured hippocampal neurons," *Neuron*, vol. 38, no. 4, pp. 611-624, 2003.

Man H. Y.,"GluA2-lacking, calcium-permeable AMPA receptors - inducers of plasticity?," *Current Opinion in Neurobiology*, vol. 21, no. 2, pp. 291-298, 2011.

Marder E. and J. M. Goaillard,"Variability, compensation and homeostasis in neuron and network function," *Nat Rev Neurosci*, vol. 7, no. 7, pp. 563-574, 2006.

Mattson M. P.,"Glutamate and neurotrophic factors in neuronal plasticity and disease," *Ann N Y Acad Sci*, vol. 1144, no., pp. 97-112, 2008.

Mazroui R., M. E. Huot, S. Tremblay, et al.,"Trapping of messenger RNA by Fragile X Mental Retardation protein into cytoplasmic granules induces translation repression," *Human Molecular Genetics*, vol. 11, no. 24, pp. 3007-3017, 2002.

Murphy DD, Rueter SM, Trojanowski JQ, Lee VM. "Synucleins are developmentally expressed, and alpha-synuclein regulates the size of the presynaptic vesicular pool in primary hippocampal neurons," *J Neurosci.* 20(9):3214-20, 2000.

Mysore S. P., C. Y. Tai, and E. M. Schuman,"N-cadherin, spine dynamics, and synaptic function," *Front Neurosci,* vol. 2, no. 2, pp. 168-175, 2008.

Nakata H. and S. Nakamura,"Brain-derived neurotrophic factor regulates AMPA receptor trafficking to post-synaptic densities via IP3R and TRPC calcium signaling," *FEBS Lett,* vol. 581, no. 10, pp. 2047-2054, 2007.

Nicoll R. A., Oliet S. H. and Malenka R. C. "NMDA receptor-dependent and metabotropic glutamate receptor-dependent forms of long-term depression coexist in CA1 hippocampal pyramidal cells," *Neurobiol Learn Mem* 70, 62-72, 1998.

Nuriya M. and R. L. Huganir,"Regulation of AMPA receptor trafficking by N-cadherin," *J Neurochem,* vol. 97, no. 3, pp. 652-661, 2006.

Ogoshi F., H. Z. Yin, Y. Kuppumbatti, et al.,"Tumor necrosis-factor-alpha (TNF-alpha) induces rapid insertion of Ca2+-permeable alpha-amino-3-hydroxyl-5-methyl-4-isoxazole-propionate (AMPA)/kainate (Ca-A/K) channels in a subset of hippocampal pyramidal neurons," *Exp Neurol,* vol. 193, no. 2, pp. 384-393, 2005.

Okuda T., L. M. Y. Yu, L. A. Cingolani, et al.,"beta-Catenin regulates excitatory postsynaptic strength at hippocampal synapses," *Proceedings of the National Academy of Sciences of the United States of America,* vol. 104, no. 33, pp. 13479-13484, 2007.

Orzylowska O., Oderfeld-Nowak B., Zaremba M., Januszewski S. and Mossakowski M. "Prolonged and concomitant induction of astroglial immu- noreactivity of interleukin-1β and interleukin-6 in the rat hippocampus after transient global ischemia," *Neuroscience Letters,* 263: 72- 76, 1999.

Papaleo F., Silverman J. L., Aney J., Tian Q., Barkan C. L., Chadman K. K., Crawley J. N. "Working memory deficits, increased anxiety-like traits, and seizure susceptibility in BDNF overexpressing mice," *Learn Mem,* 18(8):534-44, 2011.

Park S, Park JM, Kim S, Kim JA, Shepherd JD, Smith-Hicks CL, Chowdhury S, Kaufmann W, Kuhl D, Ryazanov AG, Huganir RL, Linden DJ, Worley PF. "Elongation factor 2 and fragile X mental retardation protein control the dynamic translation of Arc/Arg3.1 essential for mGluR-LTD," *Neuron.,* 59(1):70-83, 2008.

Park, M, Penick, EC, Edwards, JG, Kauer, JA, and Ehlers, MD. "Recycling endosomes supply AMPA receptors for LTP," *Science,* 305, 1972-1975, 2004.

Passafaro M., Piech V. and Sheng M. "Subunit-specific temporal and spatial patterns of AMPA receptor exocytosis in hippocampal neurons," *Nat Neurosci* 4, 917-926, 2001.

Peebles CL, Yoo J, Thwin MT, Palop JJ, Noebels JL, Finkbeiner S. "Arc regulates spine morphology and maintains network stability in vivo" *Proc Natl Acad Sci U S A*. 2010, 107(42):18173-8, 2010.

Peng P. L., X. Zhong, W. Tu, et al.,"ADAR2-dependent RNA editing of AMPA receptor subunit GluR2 determines vulnerability of neurons in forebrain ischemia," *Neuron,* vol. 49, no. 5, pp. 719-733, 2006.

Peng S., Garzon D. J., Marchese M., Klein W., Ginsberg S. D., Francis B. M., Mount H. T., Mufison E. J., Salehi A. and Fahnestock M. "BDNF mRNA is decreased in the hippocampus of individuals with Alzhemier's disease," *Neuron,* 7:695-702, 1991.

Perez-Otano and M. D. Ehlers,"Homeostatic plasticity and NMDA receptor trafficking," *Trends Neurosci,* vol. 28, no. 5, pp. 229-238, 2005.

Perry V. H., M. D. Bell, H. C. Brown, et al.,"Inflammation in the nervous system," *Curr Opin Neurobiol,* vol. 5, no. 5, pp. 636-641, 1995.

Philips H.S., Hains J. M., Amaninis M., Laramee G. R., Johnson S. A., Winslow J. W., "Decreased brain derived neurotrophic factor depends on amyloid aggregation state in transgenic mouse models of Alzheimer's disease," *J Neurosci,* 29:9321-9329, 2009.

Pisani V, Madeo G, Tassone A, Sciamanna G, Maccarrone M, Stanzione P, Pisani. "Homeostatic changes of the endocannabinoid system in Parkinson's disease," *Mov. Disord,* 26(2):216-22, 2011.

Plant K., K. A. Pelkey, Z. A. Bortolotto, et al.,"Transient incorporation of native GluR2-lacking AMPA receptors during hippocampal long-term potentiation," *Nat Neurosci,* vol. 9, no. 5, pp. 602-604, 2006.

Pozo K. and Y. Goda,"Unraveling mechanisms of homeostatic synaptic plasticity," *Neuron,* vol. 66, no. 3, pp. 337-351, 2010.

Pratt K. G., E. C. Zimmerman, D. G. Cook, et al.,"Presenilin 1 regulates homeostatic synaptic scaling through Akt signaling," *Nat Neurosci,* vol. 19, no. 9, pp. 1112-1114, 2011.

Pratt KG, Watt AJ, Griffith LC, Nelson SB, Turrigiano GG."Activity-dependent remodeling of presynaptic inputs by postsynaptic expression of activated CaMKII," *Neuron,* 39(2):269-81, 2003.

Qin Y., Y. Zhu, J. P. Baumgart, et al.,"State-dependent Ras signaling and AMPA receptor trafficking," *Genes Dev,* vol. 19, no. 17, pp. 2000-2015, 2005.

Rabinowitch I. and I. Segev,"Two opposing plasticity mechanisms pulling a single synapse," *Trends Neurosci,* vol. 31, no. 8, pp. 377-383, 2008.

Rial A. M. Verde, J. Lee-Osbourne, P. F. Worley, et al.,"Increased expression of the immediate-early gene arc/arg3.1 reduces AMPA receptor-mediated synaptic transmission," *Neuron,* vol. 52, no. 3, pp. 461-474, 2006.

Rutherford L. C., S. B. Nelson, and G. G. Turrigiano,"BDNF has opposite effects on the quantal amplitude of pyramidal neuron and interneuron excitatory synapses," *Neuron,* vol. 21, no. 3, pp. 521-30, 1998.

Saglietti L., C. Dequidt, K. Kamieniarz, et al.,"Extracellular interactions between GluR2 and N-cadherin in spine regulation," *Neuron,* vol. 54, no. 3, pp. 461-477, 2007.

Schratt G. M., E. A. Nigh, W. G. Chen, et al.,"BDNF regulates the translation of a select group of mRNAs by a mammalian target of rapamycin-phosphatidylinositol 3-kinase-dependent pathway during neuronal development," *J Neurosci,* vol. 24, no. 33, pp. 7366-7377, 2004.

Schwarz L. A., B. J. Hall, and G. N. Patrick,"Activity-dependent ubiquitination of GluA1 mediates a distinct AMPA receptor endocytosis and sorting pathway," *J Neurosci,* vol. 30, no. 49, pp. 16718-16729, 2010.

Sheng M. and Hyoung Lee S. "AMPA receptor trafficking and synaptic plasticity: major unanswered questions," *Neurosci Res* 46, 127-134, 2003.

Shepherd J. D., G. Rumbaugh, J. Wu, et al.,"Arc/Arg3.1 mediates homeostatic synaptic scaling of AMPA receptors," *Neuron,* vol. 52, no. 3, pp. 475-484, 2006.

Shi S. H., Hayashi Y., Petralia R. S., Zaman S. H., Wenthold R. J., Svoboda K. and Malinow R. "Rapid spine delivery and redistribution of AMPA receptors after synaptic NMDA receptor activation," *Science* 284, 1811-1816, 1999.

Soden M. E. and L. Chen,"Fragile X Protein FMRP Is Required for Homeostatic Plasticity and Regulation of Synaptic Strength by Retinoic Acid," *Journal of Neuroscience,* vol. 30, no. 50, pp. 16910-16921, 2010.

Song I. and Huganir R. L. "Regulation of AMPA receptors during synaptic plasticity," *Trends Neurosci* 25, 578-588, 2002.

Steinberg J. P., K. Takamiya, Y. Shen, et al.,"Targeted in vivo mutations of the AMPA receptor subunit GluR2 and its interacting protein PICK1 eliminate cerebellar long-term depression," *Neuron,* vol. 49, no. 6, pp. 845-860, 2006.

Steinmetz C. C. and G. G. Turrigiano,"Tumor necrosis factor-alpha signaling maintains the ability of cortical synapses to express synaptic scaling," *J Neurosci,* vol. 30, no. 44, pp. 14685-14690, 2010.

Stellwagen D. and R. C. Malenka,"Synaptic scaling mediated by glial TNF-alpha," *Nature*, vol. 440, no. 7087, pp. 1054-1059, 2006.

Stellwagen D., E. C. Beattie, J. Y. Seo, et al.,"Differential regulation of AMPA receptor and GABA receptor trafficking by tumor necrosis factor-alpha," *J Neurosci*, vol. 25, no. 12, pp. 3219-3228, 2005.

Steward O. and P. F. Worley,"Selective targeting of newly synthesized Arc mRNA to active synapses requires NMDA receptor activation," Neuron, vol. 30, no. 1, pp. 227-240, 2001.

Stichel CC, Augustin M, Kühn K, Zhu XR, Engels P, Ullmer C, Lübbert H. "Parkin expression in the adult mouse brain," *Eur J. Neurosci*, 12, 4181–4194, 2000.

Sutton M. A., H. T. Ito, P. Cressy, et al.,"Miniature neurotransmission stabilizes synaptic function via tonic suppression of local dendritic protein synthesis," *Cell, vol.* 125, no. 4, pp. 785-799, 2006.

Szobota S., P. Gorostiza, F. Del Bene, et al.,"Remote control of neuronal activity with a light-gated glutamate receptor," *Neuron*, vol. 54, no. 4, pp. 535-545, 2007.

Tagawa, Y., Kanold, P.O., Majdan, M. & Shatz, C.J. "Multiple periods of functional ocular dominance plasticity in mouse visual cortex," *Nat. Neurosci*, 8:380–388, 2005.

Tang T. S., E. Slow, V. Lupu, et al. "Disturbed Ca^{2+} signaling and apoptosis of medium spiny neurons in Huntington's disease," *Proc Natl Acad Sci USA*, 102: 2602–2607, 2005.

Tarkowski E., Blennow K., Wallin A. and Tarkowski A. "Intracerebral production of tumor necrosis factor-α, a local neuroprotective agent, in Alzheimer disease and vascular dementia," *J Clin Immunol*, 19: 223-230, 1999.

Terashima A., L. Cotton, K. K. Dev, et al.,"Regulation of synaptic strength and AMPA receptor subunit composition by PICK1," *J Neurosci*, vol. 24, no. 23, pp. 5381-5390, 2004.

Thiagarajan T. C., M. Lindskog, and R. W. Tsien,"Adaptation to synaptic inactivity in hippocampal neurons," *Neuron*, vol. 47, no. 5, pp. 725-737, 2005.

Tomita S., Nicoll R. A. and Bredt D. S. "PDZ protein interactions regulating glutamate receptor function and plasticity," *J Cell Biol* 153, F19-24, 2001.

Turrigiano G. G. and S. B. Nelson,"Homeostatic plasticity in the developing nervous system," *Nat Rev Neurosci*, vol. 5, no. 2, pp. 97-107, 2004.

Turrigiano G. G., K. R. Leslie, N. S. Desai, et al.,"Activity-dependent scaling of quantal amplitude in neocortical neurons," *Nature,* vol. 391, no. 6670, pp. 892-896, 1998.

Turrigiano G. G.,"The self-tuning neuron: synaptic scaling of excitatory synapses," *Cell,* vol. 135, no. 3, pp. 422-435, 2008.

Vitureira N., M. Letellier, and Y. Goda,"Homeostatic synaptic plasticity: from single synapses to neural circuits," *Curr Opin Neurobiol*, pp. 1189-1194, 2011.

Volk L., C. H. Kim, K. Takamiya, et al.,"Developmental regulation of protein interacting with C kinase 1 (PICK1) function in hippocampal synaptic plasticity and learning," *Proc Natl Acad Sci U S A,* vol. 107, no. 50, pp. 21784-21789, 2010.

Wayman G. A., Y. S. Lee, H. Tokumitsu, et al.,"Calmodulin-kinases: modulators of neuronal development and plasticity," *Neuron,* vol. 59, no. 6, pp. 914-931, 2008.

Westerman MA, Cooper-Blacketer D, Mariash A, Kotilinek L, Kawarabayashi T, Younkin LH, Carlson GA, Younkin SG and Ashe KH. "The relationship between Abeta and memory in the Tg2576 mouse model of Alzheimer's disease," *J. Neurosci,* 22, 1858–1867, 2002.

Wierenga C. J., K. Ibata, and G. G. Turrigiano,"Postsynaptic expression of homeostatic plasticity at neocortical synapses," *J Neurosci,* vol. 25, no. 11, pp. 2895-2905, 2005.

Williams M. E., S. A. Wilke, A. Daggett, et al.,"Cadherin-9 regulates synapse-specific differentiation in the developing hippocampus," *Neuron,* vol. 71, no. 4, pp. 640-655, 2011.

Wu J, Petralia RS, Kurushima H, Patel H, Jung MY, Volk L, Chowdhury S, Shepherd JD, Dehoff M, Li Y, Kuhl D, Huganir RL, Price DL, Scannevin R, Troncoso JC, Wong PC, Worley PF. "Arc/Arg3.1 regulates an endosomal pathway essential for activity-dependent β-amyloid generation," *Cell,* 147(3):615-28, 2011.

Xia J., X. Zhang, J. Staudinger, et al.,"Clustering of AMPA receptors by the synaptic PDZ domain-containing protein PICK1," *Neuron,* vol. 22, no. 1, pp. 179-187, 1999.

Yu L. M. and Y. Goda,"Dendritic signalling and homeostatic adaptation," *Curr Opin Neurobiol,* vol. 19, no. 3, pp. 327-335, 2009.

Zhang A. W., Q. M. Hou, M. Wang, et al.,"Na,K-ATPase Activity Regulates AMPA Receptor Turnover through Proteasome-Mediated Proteolysis," *Journal of Neuroscience,* vol. 29, no. 14, pp. 4498-4511, 2009.

Zhao C, Dreosti E, Lagnado L. "Homeostatic synaptic plasticity through changes in presynaptic calcium influx," *J. Neurosci,* 31(20):7492-7496, 2011.

Zhu J. J., Y. Qin, M. Zhao, et al.,"Ras and Rap control AMPA receptor trafficking during synaptic plasticity," *Cell,* vol. 110, no. 4, pp. 443-455, 2002.

Zuccato, C. et al. "Loss of huntingtin-mediated BDNF gene transcription in Huntington's disease," *Science* 293, 493–498, 2001.

In: Synaptic Plasticity
Editors: G. N. McMahon et al.
ISBN: 978-1-62081-004-0
© 2012 Nova Science Publishers, Inc.

Chapter II

ALTERNATE CALCIUM-MEDIATED SIGNALING PATHWAYS INITIATE AND LIMIT GLUTAMATERGIC PLASTICITY UNDERLYING BENZODIAZEPINE-WITHDRAWAL ANXIETY

Elizabeth I. Tietz[1,2] and Damien E. Earl[1]
[1]Departments of Physiology and Pharmacology and
[2]Neurosciences, University of Toledo College of Medicine,
Toledo OH, US

ABSTRACT

Prolonged use of benzodiazepine anxiolytics increases the likelihood of physical dependence observable as withdrawal symptoms, including anxiety. Analogous to mechanisms of synaptic plasticity underlying electrical stimulus-induced long-term potentiation, we previously identified increased synaptic insertion and subsequent calcium-calmodulin kinase Type II (CaMKII)-mediated phosphorylation of GluA1 homomeric α-amino-3-hydroxy-5-methyl-4-isoxazolepropionic acid receptors (AMPARs) as a fundamental mechanism underlying behavioral expression of anxiety. On the contrary, drug-induced sources of elevated intracellular Ca^{2+}, which may initiate AMPAR potentiation, and the mechanisms by which CaMKII is activated and deactivated may be different from those central to activity-dependent plasticity. Since L-type voltage-gated calcium channel (L-VGCC) current density doubles upon benzodiazepine withdrawal, Ca^{2+} entry through L-VGCCs, rather than N-methyl-D-aspartate receptors (NMDAR), and possibly through GluA1 homomeric AMPARs themselves may be responsible for the progressive enhancement of AMPAR function after drug removal. While Ca^{2+} influx through NMDARs is not likely involved in initiating benzodiazepine withdrawal-anxiety, a compensatory down-regulation of GluN1/GluN2B receptors, perhaps coupled with the concomitant removal of bound CaMKII limits withdrawal-anxiety expression, unlike following withdrawal from other less selective CNS depressants, such as barbiturates and ethanol. While mechanisms of GluA1 homomeric AMPAR potentiation may be highly conserved, the homeostatic regulation of CA1 neuron hyperexcitability via calcium signaling pathways differs among selective and non-selective CNS depressants associated with the severity of withdrawal symptoms and degree of physical dependence.

CONVERGENT MECHANISMS OF DRUG-INDUCED AND ACTIVITY-DEPENDENT PLASTICITY

Hippocampal CA1 pyramidal neuron excitability is governed by a homeostatic interplay between activation of inhibitory GABA-A receptors, and excitatory AMPAR and NMDAR receptors. Pyramidal cell GABA-A receptors are the main site of CNS depressant actions containing binding sites for numerous positive allosteric modulators, including benzodiazepines, neurosteroids, barbiturates, and ethanol. Benzodiazepines enhance inhibitory postsynaptic currents by enhancing GABA affinity at heteromeric GABA-A receptors containing a γ subunit thereby increasing the frequency of phasic GABA-gated chloride currents at CA1 neuronal synapses. The other allosteric modulators primarily potentiate GABA efficacy, increase the duration of single channel openings, and also enhance tonic inhibitory currents at extrasynaptic δ-containing GABA-A receptors [1,2]. CA1 neurons also express high levels of excitatory heteromeric GluA (GluR) 1–3 AMPAR subunits [3], while CA1 neuron NMDARs are composed of GluN2 (NR2) A-D subunits assembled with at least one GluN1 (NR1) subunit [4]. The effectiveness of glutamatergic, i.e. AMPAR and NMDAR antagonists to prevent withdrawal behaviors [5, 6] and our finding that increased AMPAR GluA1 subunit expression in hippocampus of chronic benzodiazepine-treated rats was tightly coupled to the expression anxiety-like behavior [7, 8] led us to explore the nature of excitatory synaptic remodeling at CA1 neuron synapses of rats treated with the water soluble benzodiazepine, flurazepam. Using this well-established model of chronic benzodiazepine treatment, our laboratory initially observed a localized, functional enhancement of glutamatergic strength at CA1 neuron Schaffer collateral synapses, i.e. an increase in the amplitude of AMPAR-mediated miniature excitatory postsynaptic currents (m)EPSCs in hippocampal slices derived from either juvenile or young adult benzodiazepine-withdrawn rats [9, 10]. The observed CA1 neuron hyperexcitability provided a neurophysiological marker of anxiety expression in the mesolimbic anxiety circuit during drug withdrawal [8, 11].

Using multidisciplinary electrophysiological, immunohistochemical and electron micrographic methodological approaches, our findings indicated that enhanced glutamate efficacy and CA1 neuron AMPAR potentiation during benzodiazepine withdrawal involves a two-step calcium (Ca^{2+})-mediated signaling process: The incorporation of comparatively few (~2-3) GluA1 homomers into CA1 neuron asymmetric synapses after 1 day resulted in significantly increased AMPAR amplitude, followed after 2 days by CaMKII-mediated GluA1Ser^{831} phosphorylation, thus increased AMPAR channel conductance [12-14]. The transient potentiation of AMPAR currents via enhanced synaptic incorporation of Ca^{2+}-permeable homomeric GluA1 AMPAR and their subsequent phosphorylation leading to enhanced channel conductance indicates that the mechanisms responsible for benzodiazepine withdrawal-induced AMPAR potentiation are very similar to those underlying activity-dependent plasticity, such as long-term potentiation (LTP) [15-17], thus may represent a final common Ca^{2+}-mediated signaling pathway mediating both drug-induced and activity-dependent plasticity.

L-VGCCs, NOT NMDARs ARE SOURCE OF ENHANCED INTRACELLULAR CALCIUM

Ca^{2+} signaling associated with synapse remodeling in models of activity-dependent plasticity at the Schaffer collateral CA1 synapse usually involves Ca^{2+} entry through NMDARs [18, 19]. However, a systemic injection of the AMPAR antagonist, GYKI-52466 (0.5mg/kg, i.p.) or the L-VGCC antagonist, nimodipine, but not the NMDA antagonist, MK-801, could reverse flurazepam withdrawal-induced AMPAR current potentiation suggesting that L-VGCC, rather than NMDAR-mediated Ca^{2+} signaling was central to benzodiazepine withdrawal-induced AMPAR potentiation (Figure 1) [7]. A striking finding in both juvenile and adult benzodiazepine-withdrawn hippocampus was a near doubling of CA1 neuron high voltage-activated (HVA) Ca^{2+} currents measured immediately upon (0 days), and up to 2 days after drug withdrawal (Figure 2) [10, 20]. The half-maximal current activation potential was negatively shifted, but steady-state inactivation was unchanged. Almost 90% of the HVA current increase in flurazepam-withdrawn neurons was blocked by 10 mM nimodipine indicating that L-VGCC-mediated currents make the primary contribution to HVA current enhancement, though a contribution from N-, P/Q-, and R-type channels cannot be ruled out. Taken together, the findings are part of a growing literature supporting a role of L-VGCCs Ca^{2+} signaling in mediating drug-induced synaptic plasticity in circuits associated with drug withdrawal symptoms, as well as addiction (for review see [21, 22]).

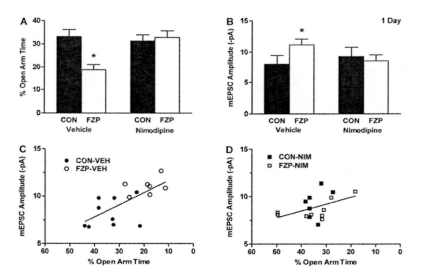

Figure 1. Effects of systemic nimodipine injection on AMPAR-mediated mEPSCs in hippocampal CA1 neurons and anxiety-like behavior during flurazepam (FZP) withdrawal. Rats injected with the L-VGCC antagonist, nimodipine (10 mg/kg, i.p.) immediately after FZP withdrawal were compared to those after vehicle injection (0.5% Tween-80, 2 ml/kg). The elevated plus-maze test was performed 1 day after nimodipine injection, followed 30 minutes later by hippocampal slice preparation and electrophysiological recording following the same protocol. (A) Open arm time in the elevated plus-maze test in 1-day FZP-withdrawn rats, 1 day after vehicle or nimodipine injection. FZP-withdrawn rats (white bars, n=9) injected with vehicle showed evidence of anxiety-like behavior, measured as a significant reduction ($p<0.05$) in the percentage of open arm time compared to control rats (black bar, n=10). There were no differences in percent open arm time between control (n=8) and FZP-withdrawn rats (n=9) after prior nimodipine injection. (B) Prior nimodipine injection averted the upregulation of AMPA receptor function 1 day after FZP withdrawal. The average

amplitudes of AMPA receptor mediated mEPSCs (V_H=-80mV) in CA1 neurons of control rats (black bar) and FZP-withdrawn rats (clear bar) were compared. The significant increase of mEPSC amplitude (*p<0.05) in CA1 neurons from FZP withdrawn (n=8 cells) compared control rats (n=8 cells) was replicated following vehicle injection. However, after prior nimodipine injection there was no difference in mEPSC amplitude in CA1 neurons from control rats (n=7 cells) vs. FZP-withdrawn rats (n=9 cells). (C) Relationship between AMPAR-mediate mEPSC amplitude in CA1 neurons and percent open arm time in individual rat that received vehicle injection. A significant positive correlation (R^2=0.4807, *P < 0.005) was found between mEPSC amplitude and percent open arm time. (D) Prior systemic nimodipine injection reversed the positive correlation between AMPAR-mediated mEPSC amplitude in CA1 neurons and open arm time percentage in the elevated plus-maze test (R^2=0.1985, p=0.0837). *Reproduced with permission from Xiang K, Tietz EI. Behav Pharmacol. 2007 Sep;18(5-6):447-60*

VGCCs are composed of a pore-forming α_1 subunit (10 subtypes) with auxiliary β and $\alpha_2\delta$ subunits (4 subtypes each). They are grouped into five classes distinguished by the unique pharmacology, gating, and conductance properties of the α_1 subunits, L- ($Ca_v1.1$-1.4), P/Q- (Cav2.1), N- (Cav2.2), R- (Cav2.3), and T-type (Cav3.1-3.3), which have different voltage activation thresholds and different physiological functions. The $Ca_v1.2$ and $Ca_v1.3$ L-VGCC α_1 subtypes expressed in neurons are selectively inhibited by dihydropyridines, phenylalkylamines, and benzothiazepines [23], the latter with structural similarities to benzodiazepines. Although $Ca_v1.2$ is four times more abundant in rat cortex and hippocampus than $Ca_v1.3$, both are expressed in the neuronal somata [24], as well as in proximal and distal dendrites near excitatory postsynapses [25-29] where they can respond to neuronal activity and mediate Ca^{2+}-dependent synaptic plasticity and changes in gene expression [30-32].

Notably, Ca^{2+} influx through L-VGCCs may also contribute to the different phases of CA1 LTP, dependent on the stimulation protocol [33, 34] or age of the animal [35]. Conditional knockout of the L-VGCC pore-forming subunit, $Ca_v1.2$ in the hippocampus and neocortex resulted in deficits in hippocampus-dependent spatial memory, probably related to the $Ca_v1.2$ channel contribution to protein synthesis-dependent late-phase LTP [36]. The contribution of L-VGCCs to some forms of LTP may be underestimated. Though application of NMDA receptor antagonists can often completely block LTP, the contribution of L-VGCCs may be missed if their activation requires additional NMDA receptor-mediated depolarization [37]. Further, the ineffectiveness of dihydropyridine antagonists to block LTP may be due to their slow inhibition of L-VGCCs when activated by brief action potential-shaped stmuli, even at high stimulus frequencies [38]. Thus, L-VGCC-mediated Ca^{2+} influx may play a prominent role in regulating glutamatergic plasticity, especially if L-VGCC function is up-regulated.

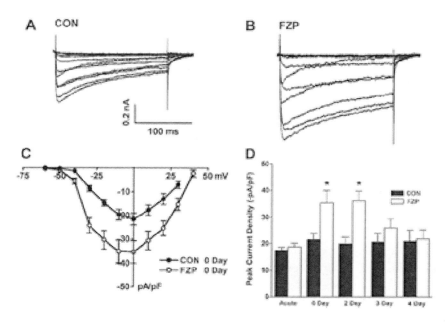

Figure 2. Doubling of HVA Ca^{2+} currents during flurazepam (FZP) withdrawal. (A, B) Representative HVA Ca^{2+} current traces elicited in neurons acutely isolated from a control (CON) and a 2-day FZP-withdrawn rat. (C) I-V relationship of HVA Ca^{2+} currents elicited from isolated CA1 neurons. Ca^{2+} currents were normalized by the membrane capacitance of individual neurons and are represented as current density (picoampere per picofarad). There was a significant increase in Ca^{2+} current density in CA1 neurons isolated from rats immediately after (0-day) withdrawal from 1-week oral FZP treatment (open circles, $n = 12$; *, $p < 0.05$), and up to 2 days (not shown, $n = 25$; *, $p < 0.05$, Student's t-test with Bonferroni's correction) compared with that from matched control rats (close circles, $n = 10$). The increase in Ca^{2+} current density was no longer significant when examined in neurons from rats withdrawn for 3 or 4 days (data not shown, $n = 7$ to 9; $p > 0.05$) compared with matched control rats ($n = 8$-10). (D) Temporal pattern of changes in CA1 neuron HVA Ca^{2+} currents after acute gavage of desalklyflurazeapm (2.5 mg/kg p.o.) or chronic FZP treatment and withdrawal. Peak Ca^{2+} current density at $V_H = 0$ mV is shown. Acute, 0 days (CON: $n = 10$, closed bars; FZP: $n = 10$, open bars); 0 days (CON: $n = 10$, closed bars; FZP: $n = 12$, open bars); 2 days (CON: $n = 25$, closed bars; FZP: $n = 25$, open bars); 3 days (CON: $n = 10$, closed bars; FZP: $n = 9$, open bars); or 4 days (CON: $n = 8$, closed bars; FZP: $n = 7$, open bars) after ending 1-week FZP treatment. *Reproduced with permission from Xiang K, Earl DE, Davis KM, Giovannucci DR, Greenfield LJ Jr, Tietz EI. J Pharmacol Exp Ther. 2008 Dec;327(3):872-83.*

L-Type Voltage Gated Calcium Channels and Withdrawal Hyperexcitability

The contribution of L-VGCC regulation to drug withdrawal symptoms was proposed in numerous studies. L-VGCC-mediated Ca^{2+} influx in hippocampal CA1 or cortical neurons is enhanced following chronic exposure to CNS depressants, including benzodiazepines [20, 39], barbiturates [40], and ethanol [41, 42] and to other drugs of abuse like nicotine [43] and cocaine [44]. Moreover, L-VGCC antagonists limit symptoms of withdrawal from benzodiazepines [7, 45], barbiturates [46], and ethanol [47]. Pierce and colleagues demonstrated that administration an L-VGCC antagonist to the nucleus accumbens shell can also attenuate reinstatement of cocaine-seeking. L-VGCC activation was further linked to downstream activation of CaMKII suggested by the increase in phospho-Thr^{286}CaMKII and phospho-Ser^{831}-GluA1 levels and increase in transport of GluA1 AMPARs to the plasma membrane [48]. Thus, the L-VGCC-dependent mechanisms of glutamatergic plasticity in nucleus accumbens induced by psychostimulants may be similar to that observed by benzodiazepines in the hippocampal CA1 region.

Increased membrane expression of L-VGCCs at asymmetric synapses could explain the enhancement of HVA currents during benzodiazepine withdrawal. An increased number of radiolabeled L-VGCC antagonist binding sites was observed on neuronal membranes following chronic exposure to various CNS depressants [39-42, 46, 47, 49] pointing to increased plasma membrane expression of $Ca_v1.2$ or $Ca_v1.3$-containing L-VGCCs as a possible mechanism mediating drug treatment-induced Ca^{2+} channel regulation. Indeed, the Ohkuma lab detected increased expression of both $Ca_v1.2$ and $Ca_v1.3$ along with $\alpha_2\delta$-1, but not β_4 subunits in cortical neurons following chronic treatment with nicotine, morphine and ethanol, as well as three benzodiazepines, administered either *in vivo* or *in vitro* [39, 42, 43, 49, 50]. Increased expression of $Ca_v1.2$ and $Ca_v1.3$ was also observed in mouse frontal cortex and limbic forebrain following chronic administration of methamphetamine, cocaine, or morphine [51]. In contrast, increased $Ca_v1.2$, but not $Ca_v1.3$ mRNA and protein expression was detected in VTA following chronic amphetamine exposure [52].

Studies from our lab indicated that CA1 neuron VGCCs activated at significantly more negative membrane potentials following chronic flurazepam treatment, which may suggest increased $Ca_v1.3$ channel function [20], in contrast to up-regulation of $Ca_v1.2$ observed in other brain regions by other drugs of abuse. Although preliminary data indicate that expression of $Ca_v1.2$ and $Ca_v1.3$ subunits was unaltered in CA1 neurons by chronic flurazepam treatment [53], regulation by post-translational modifications remains an alternate possibility, including alteration of L-VGCC function or trafficking via changes in kinase and/or phosphatase activity. Overall, the findings support a role for increased L-VGCC-mediated Ca^{2+} influx in contributing to physical dependence on a variety of drugs of abuse.

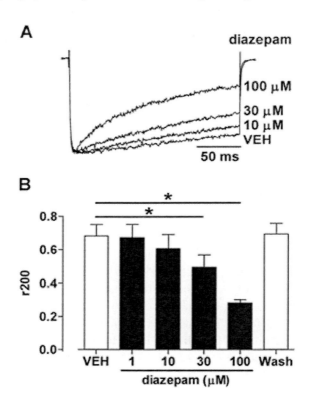

Figure 3. Diazepam enhances L-VGCC current decay. (A) Current traces were normalized to peak current. Diazepam enhanced $Ca_v1.3$ Ba^{2+} current decay during prolonged depolarization in a concentration-dependent manner. (B) The ratio of residual current at 200 ms normalized to peak current (r200 value) is shown for various diazepam concentrations. Diazepam (30 and 100 µM) significantly reduced the r200 value compared with vehicle (VEH, $n = 3$). This effect was reversed upon washout. *, $p < 0.05$, one-way ANOVA with post-hoc Dunnett's test. *Reproduced with permission from Earl DE, Tietz EI. J Pharmacol Exp Ther. 2011 Apr;337(1):301-11.*

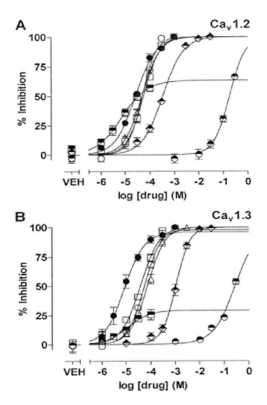

Figure 4. Concentration-response curves representing inhibition of (A) Cav1.2 and (B) Cav1.3 L-VGCCs by GABA-A receptor modulators. Diltiazem (filled circles) is shown for comparison. The rank order of potency among GABA-A receptor modulators was allopregnanolone (half-filled squares) > benzodiazepines > pentobarbital (half-filled diamonds) > ethanol (half-filled circles). The benzodiazepines tested, diazepam (open circles), flurazepam (open triangles), and desalkylflurazepam (open squares), were approximately 2- to 6-fold less potent than diltiazem. Cav1.2 and Cav1.3 L-VGCCs had similar sensitivities to inhibition by diazepam, desalkylflurazepam, allopregnanolone, and ethanol. Cav1.3 channels were 1.5-fold less sensitive to flurazepam, 3-fold less sensitive to pentobarbital, and 3-fold more sensitive to diltiazem than Cav1.2 channels. VEH represents inhibition by vehicle. Three to six cells were tested for each drug. IC50 values and Hill slopes are reported in Table 1 in [56]. *Reproduced with permission from Earl DE, Tietz EI. J Pharmacol Exp Ther. 2011 Apr;337(1):301-11.*

$Ca_v1.2$, but not $Ca_v1.3$ channels were more sensitive to the major flurazepam active metabolite, desalkylflurazepam, in a state-dependent manner, suggesting that differential allosteric modulator potency can also be observed dependent on the membrane holding potential and activation frequency [56]. State-dependent inhibition was also indicated by the ability of modulators to enhance L-VGCC current decay in a concentration-dependent manner, exemplified by diazepam in Figure 3.

Regulation of L-VGCCs during chronic drug treatment could be mediated by a direct interaction between CNS depressants and L-VGCCs [41, 54, 55]. We recently showed that various positive allosteric GABA-A receptor modulators – benzodiazepines, allopregnanolone, pentobarbital, and ethanol – can directly and concentration-dependently inhibit recombinant L-VGCCs expressed in HEK293 cells. Interestingly, $Ca_v1.2$ channels were more sensitive to inhibition by pentobarbital and flurazepam and were less sensitive to inhibition by the L-VGCC benzothiazepine antagonist, diltiazem, than $Ca_v1.3$ channels.

Concentration-response studies of GABA-A receptor allosteric modulators in recombinant L-type channels suggest that not all CNS depressants are capable of inhibiting L-VGCCs at clinically relevant concentrations (Figure 4). Thus, direct L-VGCC inhibition may play a differential role in contributing to the various neuronal adaptations that take place during chronic exposure and withdrawal from these drugs. While ethanol (IC_{50}, 300 mM) and pentobarbital (IC_{50}, 0.3 - 1 mM) directly inhibited L-VGCCs at clinically relevant concentrations, the threshold concentrations of benzodiazepines (10 µM) and allopregnanolone (3 µM) required to inhibit L-VGCCs may be too high to be clinically relevant [56]. Interestingly, the relative potencies are consistent with the comparative selectivity of these drugs for the GABA-A receptor. Ethanol is the least selective of the GABA-A allosteric modulators having the greatest number of alternate molecular targets at clinically relevant brain concentrations, followed by barbiturates, then neurosteroids and benzodiazepines, the most selective GABA-A modulator. Ethanol and barbiturate actions at various molecular targets, including L-VGCCs may also contribute to the toxic effects of these drugs, such as cognitive and memory deficits, psychomotor impairment and the potential for overdose toxicity, whereas benzodiazepines exhibit a relatively low toxicity profile [57]. Nevertheless, the acute concentration-dependent drug effects measured using recombinantly expressed L-VGCCs in HEK-293 cells may not represent what occurs during chronic drug exposure of native channels expressed in cultured neurons or *in vivo*. Notably, we also observed a significant concentration- and use-dependent inhibition of VGCCs following preincubation of cultured hippocampal neurons with flurazepam at concentrations (≤1 µM) measured in rat brain homogenates during chronic treatment (Figure 5) [20].

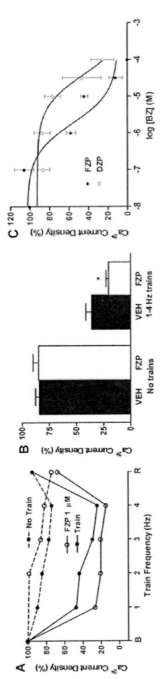

Figure 5. Use- and concentration-dependent inhibition of high voltage activated (HVA) Ca^{2+} current by benzodiazepines. The use- and concentration-dependent effect of benzodiazepines on HVA Ca^{2+} currents were evaluated in DIV 10 to 14 hippocampal cultured cells using whole-cell techniques. (A) Use-dependent effect of flurazepam (FZP) on HVA Ca^{2+} currents. The Ca^{2+} current density was normalized and expressed as the percentage of the current evoked by baseline test pulse. Without a train of consecutive depolarizing pulses, 1 μM FZP showed little inhibitory effect on HVA Ca^{2+} current. Following depolarizing stimulus train application at frequencies of 1, 2, 3, or 4 Hz, preincubation with 1 μM FZP resulted in approximately 45% inhibition by of HVA Ca^{2+} current density compared with that in the presence of vehicle. Note the Ca^{2+}-dependent inactivation of HVA Ca^{2+} current after trains of consecutive depolarizing pulses. A recovery test pulse (R), without prior train stimulation was given at the end of the recording to exclude run-down of Ca^{2+} channel function or seal degradation. (B) Mean inhibition of HVA Ca^{2+} current by FZP. FZP (1 μM) had no effect on HVA Ca^{2+} currents in hippocampal cultured neurons in which depolarizing pulses were not applied (no trains: VEH, solid bar; FZP, open bar; $p > 0.05$). In neurons in which consecutive depolarizing trains were applied, 1 μM FZP inhibited 45% of HVA Ca^{2+} currents, which was similar across all frequencies sampled; therefore, these data were averaged [1–4-Hz trains: Vehicle (VEH), $n = 4$; FZP, $n = 4$; $*p < 0.05$, Student's t-test]. (C) Concentration-dependent inhibition of HVA Ca^{2+} current by benzodiazepines. FZP and diazepam (DZP, 0.1–100 μM) effects to inhibit Ca^{2+} current test pulses were evaluated after 5-min preincubation. Ca^{2+} current density was normalized and expressed as the percentage of the current evoked in the presence of vehicle. *Reproduced with permission from Xiang K, Earl DE, Davis KM, Giovannucci DR, Greenfield LJ Jr, Tietz EI. J Pharmacol Exp Ther. 2008 Dec;327(3):872-83.*

Enhanced L-VGCC function following chronic benzodiazepine exposure may also occur via other indirect interactions. For example, benzodiazepines enhance GABA-A receptor-mediated hyperpolarization to reduce neuronal activity, which could also reduce neuronal L-VGCC activity, an in-turn lead to homeostatic up-regulation of calcium channels. On the contrary, it is also possible that the benzodiazepine-GABA-A receptor interaction increased L-VGCC-mediated Ca^{2+} influx during flurazepam treatment, since we also observed a GABA-A receptor-mediated depolarization in CA1 neurons during flurazepam withdrawal [58, 59], yet it is unknown whether the depolarization exists during treatment. Preliminary experiments have not detected any alteration in expression of the cation-chloride co-transporter KCC2 in flurazepam-withdrawn CA1 homogenates (data not shown). However, reduced activity of KCC2 or increased activity of NKCC1 cannot be ruled out, either of which could cause an intracellular Cl^- accumulation and explain the significant depolarizing shift in the GABA-A receptor reversal potential during flurazepam withdrawal [60] correlating with the GABA-A receptor-mediated depolarization. Clearly, additional studies are needed to decipher the complex regulation of ion channels by benzodiazepines, keeping in mind the importance of network activity *in vivo*.

NMDA RECEPTOR DOWNREGULATION SECONDARY TO AMPAR POTENTIATION

The heightened VGCC-mediated Ca^{2+} entry during benzodiazepine withdrawal and the ability of pre-injection of nimodipine, rather than MK-801 to block anxiety indicated that L-VGCCs, rather than NMDARs may mediate downstream Ca^{2+}-mediated AMPAR potentiation. On the other hand, the finding that GYKI-52466 preinjection could prevent the protracted decline in NMDAR function suggested that the observed regulation of NMDAR was compensatory, rather than central to enhanced AMPAR strength and that downregulation of NMDAR function may instead serve a protective, negative-feedback role to prevent AMPAR-mediated neuronal over-excitation [7, 8, 61].

NMDAR surface expression is dynamically regulated by membrane insertion [62, 63], lateral diffusion and internalization [64-66], and by various kinases, including CaMKII [67-69]. Since our earlier *in situ* hybridization studies had identified a reduction in GluN2B mRNA [61], we proposed that a pool of NMDARs containing GluN2B subunits might be regulated at CA1 synapses. Consistent with previous findings [61] reduced GluN1 and GluN2B, but not GluN2A subunit levels, were observed in immunoblots of PSD-enriched subfractions of CA1 minislices from 2-day, but not 1-day, flurazepam-withdrawn rats. We also examined whether CaMKII-mediated phosphorylation of GluN2B subunits might play a role in NMDAR regulation during benzodiazepine withdrawal by probing the levels of expression of the CaMKII substrate, phospho-Ser^{1303}GluN2B subunit and its ratio to total GluN2B subunit levels. However, neither phospho-Ser^{1303}GluN2B levels nor ratios were changed during drug withdrawal [70].

Another kinase, casein kinase 2 (CK2) phosphorylates Ser^{1480}GluN2B within the C-terminal PDZ ligand domain, disrupts GluN2B, PSD-95 and SAP102 interactions and also results in decreased GluN2B surface expression. Thus, we also predicted that phosphorylation of Ser^{1480}GluN2B in 1- or 2-day flurazepam-withdrawn rats may be increased and evaluated CK2 activity and Ser^{1480}GluN2B immunolevels. On the contrary, CK2 activity, but not CK2α expression decreased in 2-day, but not 1-day PSD subfractions suggesting decreased CK2 activity may instead be a compensatory response to GluN2B downregulation (unpublished observations). Although phospho-Ser^{1480}GluN2B and GluN2B were both significantly ($p<.05$) downregulated after 2 days, the phospho-ratio was unchanged.

Quantitative EM studies provided direct evidence that depression of NMDAR function involved negative modulation of GluN1/GluN2B receptors [71]. As with the GluA1 subunits, the spatial localization of immunogold particles associated with NMDAR subunits was consistent with a predominantly postsynaptic localization. GluN1- and GluN2B-immunogold density and the percentage of immunopositive synapses were significantly reduced in CA1 tissues from flurazepam-withdrawn rats (Figures 6 and 7). On the contrary, the density and perentage of synapses labeled with the GluN2A subunit antibody were unaltered. These findings provided solid evidence for reduced synaptic GluN1/GluN2B receptors in the CA1 SR region during BZ withdrawal, while GluN1/GluN2A receptor numbers were preserved. There was no evidence of lateral displacement of GluN2B subunits in 2-day flurazepam-withdrawn tissues, though we cannot rule out that GluN1/GluN2B NMDAR did not move through the lateral synaptic compartment.

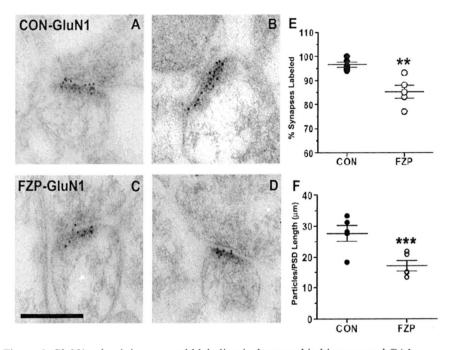

Figure 6. GluN1 subunit immunogold labeling is decreased in hippocampal CA1 asymmetric synapses during FZP withdrawal. (A, B) Representative electron micrographs of GluN1-subunit immunogold labeling in hippocampal CA1 stratum radiatum from control tissues. Immunogold particles (10 nm) are located primarily within the PSD and some particles extend into the synaptic cleft. (C, D) Representative images of GluN1-labeled asymmetric synapses from FZP-withdrawn tissues show similar distribution of immunogold labeling. (E) The percentage of synapses with immunogold labeling for GluN1 (containing at least one immunogold particle) was significantly reduced (**$P < 0.01$, Student's t-test) in synapses from FZP-withdrawn rats (white dots) compared to controls (black dots). Each dot represents the average obtained from a single animal (n = 50 to 71 synapses per animal). The average for all animals (large horizontal bar) and standard error of the mean (SEM, smaller bars) are superimposed to the dotplots (n = 5 animals). (F) GluN1 immunogold density estimated by the number of gold particles per micron synaptic length was also notably reduced in synapses from FZP-withdrawn rats (white dots) compared to controls (black dots) (n = 5 rats/group, ***$P = 0.009$, MANOVA). As above, average ± SEM for all five animals is superimposed in the aligned dotplot. All images are at the same magnification. Scale bar = 0.25 µm. *Reproduced with permission from Das P, Zerda R, Alvarez FJ, Tietz EI. J Comp Neurol. 2010 Nov 1;518(21):4311-28.*

We next explored the functional consequence of the significant reduction in synaptic NMDA receptors and NMDA-elicited currents [61, 70, 71]. We observed that superfusion of the GluN2B-selective antagonist, ifenprodil eliminated the reduction in NMDAR-mediated evoked currents (Figure 8) further implicating the downregulation of GluN2B-containing NMDARs in halting the progression of withdrawal-anxiety [70]. GluN1/GluN2B NMDAR carry more charge per single synaptic event than GluN1/GluN2A NMDAR [72] and introduce more Ca^{2+} influx per unit current [73]. Therefore, removal of GluN2B-containing NMDAR may more efficiently reduce abnormal levels of Ca^{2+} influx and the consequent effects on downstream signaling cascades.

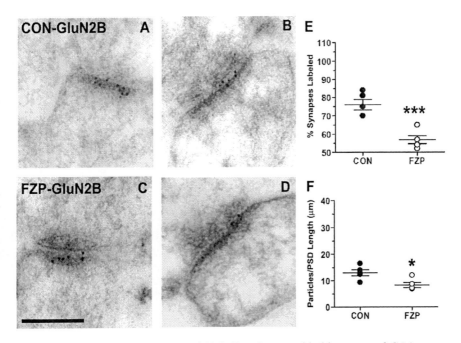

Figure 7. GluN2B subunit immunogold labeling decreased in hippocampal CA1 asymmetric synapses during FZP withdrawal. (A, B) Representative electron micrographs of GluN2B-labeled asymmetric synapses from control and (C, D) FZP-withdrawn synapses show 10 nm immunogold particles mainly in the postsynaptic density and extending into the synaptic cleft. E) FZP-withdrawal caused a significant reduction in the total percentage of synapses labeled with at least one immunogold particle compared to controls (***P < 0.001, Student's *t*-test) and (F) in mean immunogold density (n 1/4 5 rats/group, *P < 0.014, MANOVA). As in Figure 6, each dot represents a single animal average (43–59 synapses analyzed in each animal) with the total five animals average and SEM superimposed. All images are at the same magnification. Scale bar = 0.25 μm. *Reproduced with permission from Das P, Zerda R, Alvarez FJ, Tietz EI. J Comp Neurol. 2010 Nov 1;518(21):4311-28.*

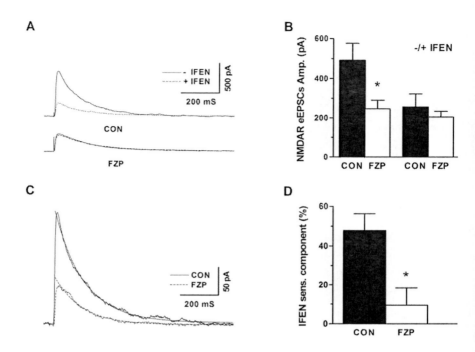

Figure 8. Reduction in GluN2B-mediated eEPSCs in CA1 neurons from 2-day FZP-withdrawn rats. **(A)** Representative traces recorded before (solid line) and after (dotted line) application of 1 µM ifenprodil, a GluN2B subunit-selective antagonist. **(B)** The amplitude of NMDAR-mediated evoked EPSCs was decreased in CA1 neurons from 2-day FZP-withdrawn rats, an effect abolished by ifenprodil. **(C)** A single-exponential decay fit of mean ifenprodil-sensitive current revealed a similar decay time-constant (CON: t=0.15 sec vs. FZP: t=0.14 sec, * p<0.05). **(D)** The amplitude of the ifenprodil-sensitive component was significantly decreased in neurons from 2-day FZP-withdrawn rats, while the non-GluN2B component was not different between experimental groups. *Reproduced with permission from Shen G, Tietz EI. J Pharmacol Exp Ther. 2011 Jan;336(1):265-73.*

Additional electrophysiological studies in which total CA1 neuron current output was measured as total charge transfer indicated that the significant depression of currents mediated by downregulation of GluN2B-containing NMDAR could indeed offset AMPAR potentiation due to recruitment and phosphorylation of GluA1 homomers at CA1 synapses. That is, the total charge transfer in mixed currents mediated by both AMPA and NMDA receptors was not different between neurons from either experimental group indicating that CA1 neuron hyperexcitability, a marker for the expression of anxiety was normalized by GluN1/GluN2B downregulation (Figure 9) [8, 70].

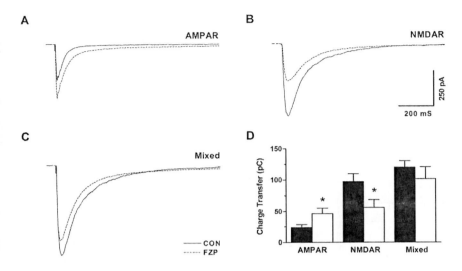

Figure 9. AMPA preincubation induced GluN2B-mediated NMDAR downregulation in slices from 1-day FZP-withdrawn rats. (A) Incubation (30 min) of hippocampal slices in 1 µM AMPA resulted in decreased NMDAR-mediated eEPSC amplitude in CA1 neurons from 1-day FZP-withdrawn rats, as in 2-day FZP-withdrawn rats, but not in neurons from control rats. (B) Blockade of GluN2B-containing NMDAR with ifenprodil diminished the effect of AMPA incubation in slices from 1-day FZP-withdrawn rats. (C) Average traces of ifenprodil-sensitive currents in slices from control -AMPA (solid black line), control +AMPA (solid gray line), 1-day FZP -AMPA (black dotted line) and 1-day FZP +AMPA (gray dotted line) indicated that AMPA incubation promoted a decrease in GluN2B-containing NMDAR currents in 1-day FZP-withdrawn rats. (D) The ifenprodil-sensitive component was significantly decreased in slices from 1-day FZP-withdrawn rats preincubated with AMPA. *Reproduced with permission from Shen G, Tietz EI. J Pharmacol Exp Ther. 2011 Jan;336(1):265-73.*

Since CaMKII levels were increased we propose that an enhanced protein-protein interaction between GluN2B could result in autonomous, Ca^{2+}/calmodulin-independent activity as shown by Bayer et al. [74, 75] and may explain our observation of enhanced GluA1Ser^{831} phosphorylation in the absence of an enhancement of phospho-Thr^{286}CaMKII levels. Alternatively, enhanced Ca^{2+} influx through both L-VGCCs and Ca^{2+}-permeable GluA1 homomeric AMPARs may increase the activity of CaMKII localized to the PSD via binding to GluN2B. Decreased synaptic incorporation or enhanced endocytosis of GluN2B-NMDAR could then serve as one mechanism for CaMKII removal and the return of AMPAR synaptic strength to basal levels. Preliminary studies show that CaMKII levels may actually be reduced at CA1 asymmetric synapses in tissues in which GluN1/GluN2B receptors are also reduced [53]. Removal of GluN1/GluN2B receptors and/or removal of CaMKII would thus no longer permit AMPAR phosphorylation, eventually halting AMPAR potentiation and anxiety as observed on day 3 of withdrawal [8, 13, 70].

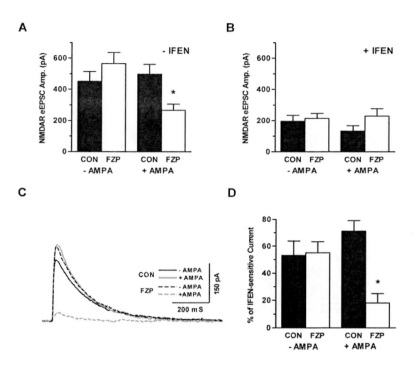

Figure 10. Depression of NMDAR current counteracted AMPAR potentiation in CA1 neurons from 2-day FZP-withdrawn rats. (A-C) Average traces of eEPSCs recorded in ACSF without Mg^{2+} at V_H=-40mV using a stimulus intensity to elicit a half-maximal response. The charge transfer of mixed current mediated by both AMPAR and NMDAR was not different between neurons from control (120.0 ± 10.2 pC, n=7) and 2-day FZP-withdrawn (101.7 ± 18.8 pC, n=7, p = 0.4099) rats. (A) AMPAR-mediated charge transfer dissected using APV, increased in neurons from 2-day FZP-withdrawn rats (CON, 23.5 ± 4.7 pC vs. FZP, 46.5 ± 9.0 pC, n=7, p = 0.04024). (B) In contrast, charge transfer mediated by NMDAR showed a significant decrease in neurons from 2-day FZP-withdrawn rats (CON, 97.2 ± 16.7 pC vs. FZP 56.4 ± 12.7 pC, n=7, p = 0.0419). (C) Charge transfer mediated by mixed AMPAR and NMDAR currents was unchanged in CA1 neurons from 2-day FZP-withdrawn rats reflecting the increased AMPAR-mediated and decreased NMDAR-mediated charge transfer. (* p<0.05). *Reproduced with permission from Shen G, Tietz EI. J Pharmacol Exp Ther. 2011 Jan;336(1):265-73.*

Activation of Ca^{2+}-permeable GluA1 homomers may additionally contribute to NMDAR downregulation and may also affect downstream NMDAR-CaMKII interactions. Therefore, we tested whether AMPA activation of newly inserted GluA1 homomers could modulate NMDAR function. Indeed, preincubation (0.5 h) of hippocampal slices with 1 µM AMPA induced a significant reduction in NMDAR currents in 1-day flurazepam-withdrawn rats (Figure 10), a withdrawal time-point when a reduction in evoked NMDA currents were previously undetectable [8]. These findings implied that additional Ca^{2+} influx through activation of recently incorporated Ca^{2+}-permeable GluA1 homomeric AMPARs might also play an important role to induce downregulation of NMDAR function and possibly NMDAR-CaMKII interactions [67, 67, 74, 75].

PHYSIOLOGICAL HOMEOSTATIC BRAKE TO LESSEN BENZODIAZEPINE-WITHDRAWAL ANXIETY

In contrast to the potentially life-threatening symptoms observed following the abrupt withdrawal from ethanol or barbiturates, benzodiazepine withdrawal symptoms are comparably modest. In benzodiazepine-withdrawn rats anxiety was not observed 2-days after drug withdrawal due to NMDAR downregulation. Our studies provide strong evidence that this represents a homeostatic brake on the hyperexcitability in the limbic anxiety circuit. During the period of CA1 neuron hyperexcitability attributable to enhanced AMPAR-mediated glutamatergic strength, a the compensatory decrease in GluN1/GluN2B receptor expression and function occurs that normalizes CA1 neuron output and cuts short the expression of anxiety [8, 70, 71, 76].

Quite the opposite of our finding that the number of synaptic GluN1/GluN2B receptors was reduced following prolonged benzodiazepine administration, an increased number of NMDAR ligand binding sites was observed in several brain areas following chronic ethanol or barbiturate treatment, whereas kainate and AMPAR ligand binding sites were decreased, respectively [77, 78]. NMDAR function was consistently enhanced in the amygdala following chronic ethanol exposure *in vivo* [79] and in cerebellar and cortical neurons *in vitro* [77, 80]. In particular, upregulation of GluN2B mRNA and protein levels was detected following chronic or chronic intermittent ethanol exposure *in vivo* and *in vitro* [81-84], suggesting that as opposed to benzodiazepine withdrawal, upregulation of GluN2B-containing

NMDARs may underlie the intense, often life-threatening ethanol withdrawal symptoms. The variability in glutamatergic regulation by GABA-A receptor modulators may be due to the different molecular targets of these compounds, as both ethanol and barbiturates inhibit NMDARs [85, 86], which may promote the up-regulation of this excitatory receptor class during drug withdrawal. Thus, the NMDAR, especially those containing the GluN2B subunit, may be a potential therapeutic target to ameliorate drug withdrawal symptoms associated with several classes of CNS depressants.

CONVERGENCE AND DIVERGENCE OF MECHANISMS OF ACTIVITY AND DRUG-INDUCED PLASTICITY

As shown in our overall model of benzodiazepine withdrawal-anxiety plasticity mechanisms (Figure 11), both the convergent and divergent signaling mechanisms uncovered during benzodiazepine withdrawal may also be central to neuronal plasticity associated with dependence and addiction to various drugs of abuse [47, 48, 87-93], including benzodiazepines [94]. The transient potentiation of AMPAR currents via enhanced synaptic incorporation of Ca^{2+}-permeable homomeric GluA1 AMPAR is a consistent finding among models of activity-dependent plasticity, such as LTP [15-17, 95] and drug-induced plasticity [48, 87, 90, 92, 96, 97]. Upregulation of L-VGCCs has also been described with chronic ethanol, nicotine and morphine, and more recently, several benzodiazepines [39, 43, 50, 98, 99].

Our novel finding that synaptic insertion and subsequent CaMKII-mediated Ser^{831} phosphorylation of GluA1 homomers contributes to benzodiazepine withdrawal-induced AMPAR potentiation may represent a final common pathway mediating both drug-induced and activity-dependent plasticity [10]. Moreover, here we summarize data that suggests that mechanisms upstream of CaMKII activation which initiate AMPAR potentiation may differ between models of activity-dependent plasticity, such as LTP which results from brief, coincident activation of excitatory pathways vs. drug-induced plasticity, which results from more persistent, selective activation of drug targets in specific neural circuits. While NMDARs are typically the source of Ca^{2+} for AMPAR potentiation in the former models, Ca^{2+} influx through L-VGCCs may play a more prominent role in drug-induced glutamatergic plasticity.

Alternate Calcium-Mediated Signaling Pathways Initiate ... 63

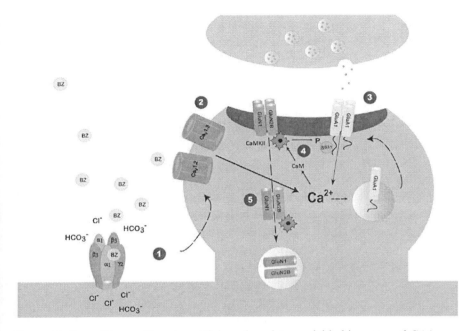

Figure 11. Overall benzodiazepine withdrawal-anxiety model in hippocampal CA1 neurons. **1:** Persistent benzodiazepine allosteric enhancement of the inhibitory GABA-A receptor leads to a bicarbonate ion-dependent GABA-mediated depolarization [59] and **2:** enhanced L-VGCC activation, as well as a doubling of Ca^{2+} current density [20]. Since both AMPAR potentiation and benzodiazepine withdrawal-anxiety were prevented by systemic pre-injection of either an AMPAR antagonist or an L-VGCC blocker, but not an NMDAR antagonist [7, 8], we propose that increased Ca^{2+} influx through L-VGCCs initiates **3:** an increase in glutamate efficacy via synaptic insertion of Ca^{2+}-permeable GluA1 homomeric AMPARs and increased AMPAR current amplitude at CA1 synapses of 1-day FZP-withdrawn rats [12, 13, 101]. This is followed after 2 days by **4:** CaMKII-mediated Ser^{831} phosphorylation of GluA1 homomers and increased AMPAR current conductance analogous to mechanisms of activity-dependent AMPAR potentiation [13, 16, 17, 76]. **5:** NMDAR function and expression is decreased secondary to AMPAR potentiation [7, 8]. Our studies indicate that the numbers of NMDAR numbers are downregulated in the CA1 synapse [61, 70, 71] by decreased insertion and/or removal of CA1 neuron GluN1/GluN2B NMDARs. Since CaMKII binds to the GluN2B subunit [67,68], GluN2B downregulation may end CaMKII-mediated Ser^{831} phosphorylation of GluA1 homomers and restore AMPAR currents to basal levels after 4 days [8]. In the meanwhile, decreased numbers of synaptic GluN1/GluN2BRs normalize CA1 neuron total charge transfer to mitigate the effects of AMPAR current potentiation in FZP-withdrawn rats [70], and serve as the initial physiological brake to limit CA1 neuron hyperexcitability and benzodiazepine withdrawal-anxiety. *Reproduced with permission from Das P, Zerda R, Alvarez FJ, Tietz EI. J Comp Neurol. 2010 Nov 1;518(21):4311-28.*

On the contrary as we have noted, similar mechanisms involving CaMKII-mediated GluA1 homomer incorporation and phosphorylation have been described in CA1 neurons in our benzodiazepine-withdrawal model and in dopamine neurons in accumbens in relation to reinstatement of cocaine-seeking. Interestingly, L-VGCCs were also the source of Ca^{2+} entry responsible for CaMKII-mediated effects on reinstatement of cocaine seeking since the effect was prevented by diltiazem [48]. Unlike with benzodiazepine withdrawal, levels of phospho-Thr^{286}CaMKII were elevated in the latter model. Nevertheless, the finding that the latter model of drug relapse also shares this common mechanism of Ca^{2+} entry suggests that this fundamental commonality might be more broadly therapeutically exploited to diminish dependence and addictive behaviors often seen with drug abuse, in particular for polydrug abusers who often abuse benzodiazepines [100].

ACKNOWLEDGEMENTS

The authors would like to acknowledge the intellectual and technical contributions from the co-authors of the work cited including: Drs. Paromita Das, L. John, Greenfield Jr., Francisco J. Alvarez, David R. Giovannucci, William T. Gunning, III, Ricardo Zerda, Guofu Shen, Kun Xiang, Jun Song, Scott M. Lilly, Bradley J. Van Sickle. The authors are appreciative of the contributions of Kathleen M. Davis, Angela S. Cox, and Kathryn Schak. The authors also thank of Alexandrea Wenzlaff, Krista Petee, Margarete Otting and William Ferencak, III for their expert technical assistance. Additional acknowledgements can be found within the published reports. The studies described were funded by department of Health and Human Services Grants from the National Institute on Drug Abuse to EI Tietz: RO1-DA04075-15; RO1-DA018341-05; DE Earl: F30-DA026675; SM Lilly: F30-DA06041-01; and BJ Van Sickle: F30-DA14142.

REFERENCES

[1] Uusi-Oukari, M; Korpi, ER. Regulation of GABA(A) receptor subunit expression by pharmacological agents. *Pharmacol. Rev.*, 2010, 62, 97-135.

[2] Olsen, RW; Sieghart, W. GABA A receptors: subtypes provide diversity of function and pharmacology. *Neuropharmacology*, 2009, 56, 141-148.

[3] Wenthold, RJ; Petralia, RS; Blahos, JII; Niedzielski, AS. Evidence for multiple AMPA receptor complexes in hippocampal CA1/CA2 neurons. *J. Neurosci.*, 1996, 16, 1982-1989.

[4] Blahos, Jn; Wenthold, RJ. Relationship between N-methyl-D-aspartate receptor NR1 splice variants and NR2 subunits. *J. Biol. Chem.*, 1996, 271, 15669-15674.

[5] Steppuhn, KG; Turski, L. Diazepam dependence prevented by glutamate antagonists. *Proc. Natl. Acad. Sci. USA*, 1993, 90, 6889-6893.

[6] Allison, C; Pratt, JA. Neuroadaptive processes in GABAergic and glutamatergic systems in benzodiazepine dependence. *Pharmacol. Ther.*, 2003, 98, 171-195.

[7] Xiang, K; Tietz, EI. Benzodiazepine-induced hippocampal CA1 neuron alpha-amino-3-hydroxy-5-methylisoxasole-4-propionic acid (AMPA) receptor plasticity linked to severity of withdrawal anxiety: differential role of voltage-gated calcium channels and N-methyl-D-aspartic acid receptors. *Behav. Pharmacol.*, 2007, 18, 447-460.

[8] Van Sickle, BJ; Xiang, K; Tietz, EI. Transient plasticity of hippocampal CA1 neuron glutamate receptors contributes to benzodiazepine withdrawal-anxiety. *Neuropsychopharmacology*, 2004, 29, 1994-2006.

[9] Van Sickle, B; Tietz, E. Selective enhancement of AMPA receptor-mediated function in hippocampal CA1 neurons from chronic benzodiazepine-treated rats. *Neuropharmacology*, 2002, 43, 11-27.

[10] Tietz, EI; Earl, DE. Calcium-calmodulin kinase Type II-mediated glutamatergic plasticity underlies expression of benzodiazepine-withdrawal anxiety. Glutamate: Functions, Regulation and Disorders. New York, NY: Nova Science Publishers, Inc.; in press.

[11] McNaughton, N; Gray, JA. Anxiolytic action on the behavioural inhibition system implies multiple types of arousal contribute to anxiety. *J. Affect. Disord.*, 2000, 61, 161-176.

[12] Song, J; Shen, G; Greenfield, LJJ; Tietz, EI. Benzodiazepine Withdrawal-Induced Glutamatergic Plasticity Involves Up-Regulation of GluR1-Containing {alpha}-Amino-3-hydroxy-5-methylisoxasole-4-propionic Acid Receptors in Hippocampal CA1 Neurons. *J. Pharmacol. Exp. Ther.*, 2007, 322, 569-581.

[13] Shen, G; Van Sickle, BJ; Tietz, EI. Calcium/calmodulin-dependent protein kinase II mediates hippocampal glutamatergic plasticity during

benzodiazepine withdrawal. *Neuropsychopharmacology*, 2010, 35, 1897-1909.
[14] Oh, MC; Derkach, VA. Dominant role of the GluR2 subunit in regulation of AMPA receptors by CaMKII. *Nat. Neurosci.*, 2005, 8, 853-854.
[15] Plant, K; Pelkey, KA; Bortolotto, ZA et al. Transient incorporation of native GluR2-lacking AMPA receptors during hippocampal long-term potentiation. *Nat. Neurosci.*, 2006, 9, 602-604.
[16] Guire, ES; Oh, MC; Soderling, TR; Derkach, VA. Recruitment of calcium-permeable AMPA receptors during synaptic potentiation is regulated by CaM-kinase I. *J. Neurosci.*, 2008, 28, 6000-6009.
[17] Derkach, VA; Oh, MC; Guire, ES; Soderling, TR. Regulatory mechanisms of AMPA receptors in synaptic plasticity. *Nat. Rev. Neurosci.*, 2007, 8, 101-113.
[18] Collingridge, GL; Isaac, JT; Wang, YT. Receptor trafficking and synaptic plasticity. *Nat. Rev. Neurosci.*, 2004, 5, 952-962.
[19] Tsien, JZ; Huerta, PT; Tonegawa, S. The essential role of hippocampal CA1 NMDA receptor-dependent synaptic plasticity in spatial memory. *Cell*, 1996, 87, 1327-1338.
[20] Xiang, K; Earl, DE; Davis, KM; Giovannucci, DR; Greenfield, LJJ; Tietz, EI. Chronic benzodiazepine administration potentiates high voltage-activated calcium currents in hippocampal CA1 neurons. *J. Pharmacol. Exp. Ther.*, 2008, 327, 872-883.
[21] Licata, SC; Pierce, RC. The roles of calcium/calmodulin-dependent and Ras/mitogen-activated protein kinases in the development of psychostimulant-induced behavioral sensitization. *J. Neurochem.*, 2003, 85, 14-22.
[22] Rajadhyaksha, AM; Kosofsky, BE. Psychostimulants, L-type calcium channels, kinases, and phosphatases. *Neuroscientist*, 2005, 11, 494-502.
[23] Catterall, WA; Perez-Reyes, E; Snutch, TP; Striessnig, J. International Union of Pharmacology. XLVIII. Nomenclature and structure-function relationships of voltage-gated calcium channels. *Pharmacol. Rev.*, 2005, 57, 411-425.
[24] Hell, JW; Westenbroek, RE; Warner, C et al. Identification and differential subcellular localization of the neuronal class C and class D L-type calcium channel alpha 1 subunits. *J. Cell Biol.*, 1993, 123, 949-962.
[25] Obermair, GJ; Szabo, Z; Bourinet, E; Flucher, BE. Differential targeting of the L-type Ca^{2+} channel alpha 1C (CaV1.2) to synaptic and

extrasynaptic compartments in hippocampal neurons. *Eur. J. Neurosci.*, 2004, 19, 2109-2122.
[26] Day, M; Wang, Z; Ding, J et al. Selective elimination of glutamatergic synapses on striatopallidal neurons in Parkinson disease models. *Nat. Neurosci.*, 2006, 9, 251-259.
[27] Tippens, AL; Pare, JF; Langwieser, N et al. Ultrastructural evidence for pre- and postsynaptic localization of Cav1.2 L-type Ca^{2+} channels in the rat hippocampus. *J. Comp. Neurol.*, 2008, 506, 569-583.
[28] Leitch, B; Szostek, A; Lin, R; Shevtsova, O. Subcellular distribution of L-type calcium channel subtypes in rat hippocampal neurons. *Neuroscience*, 2009, 164, 641-657.
[29] Zhang, M; Moller, M; Broman, J; Sukiasyan, N; Wienecke, J; Hultborn, H. Expression of calcium channel CaV1.3 in cat spinal cord: light and electron microscopic immunohistochemical study. *J. Comp. Neurol.*, 2008, 507, 1109-1127.
[30] Striessnig, J; Koschak, A; Sinnegger-Brauns, MJ et al. Role of voltage-gated L-type Ca^{2+} channel isoforms for brain function. *Biochem. Soc. Trans.*, 2006, 34, 903-909.
[31] Dolmetsch, RE; Pajvani, U; Fife, K; Spotts, JM; Greenberg, ME. Signaling to the nucleus by an L-type calcium channel-calmodulin complex through the MAP kinase pathway. *Science*, 2001, 294, 333-339.
[32] Barbado, M; Fablet, K; Ronjat, M; De Waard, M. Gene regulation by voltage-dependent calcium channels. *Biochim. Biophys. Acta.*, 2009, 1793, 1096-1104.
[33] Grover, LM; Teyler, TJ. Different mechanisms may be required for maintenance of NMDA receptor-dependent and independent forms of long-term potentiation. *Synapse*, 1995, 19, 121-133.
[34] Morgan, SL; Teyler, TJ. Electrical stimuli patterned after the theta-rhythm induce multiple forms of LTP. *J. Neurophysiol.*, 2001, 86, 1289-1296.
[35] Shankar, S; Teyler, TJ; Robbins, N. Aging differentially alters forms of long-term potentiation in rat hippocampal area CA1. *J. Neurophysiol.*, 1998, 79, 334-341.
[36] Moosmang, S; Haider, N; Klugbauer, N et al. Role of hippocampal Cav1.2 Ca^{2+} channels in NMDA receptor-independent synaptic plasticity and spatial memory. *J. Neurosci.*, 2005, 25, 9883-9892.
[37] Morgan, SL; Teyler, TJ. VDCCs and NMDARs underlie two forms of LTP in CA1 hippocampus in vivo. *J. Neurophysiol.*, 1999, 82, 736-740.

[38] Helton, TD; Xu, W; Lipscombe, D. Neuronal L-type calcium channels open quickly and are inhibited slowly. *J. Neurosci.*, 2005, 25, 10247-10251.

[39] Katsura, M; Shibasaki, M; Kurokawa, K; Tsujimura, A; Ohkuma, S. Up-regulation of L-type high voltage-gated calcium channel subunits by sustained exposure to 1,4- and 1,5-benzodiazepines in cerebrocortical neurons. *J. Neurochem.*, 2007, 103, 2518-2528.

[40] Rabbani, M; Little, HJ. Increases in neuronal Ca^{2+} flux after withdrawal from chronic barbiturate treatment. *Eur. J. Pharmacol.*, 1999, 364, 221-227.

[41] Messing, RO; Carpenter, CL; Diamond, I; Greenberg, DA. Ethanol regulates calcium channels in clonal neural cells. *Proc. Natl. Acad. Sci. USA*, 1986, 83, 6213-6215.

[42] Katsura, M; Shibasaki, M; Hayashida, S; Torigoe, F; Tsujimura, A; Ohkuma, S. Increase in expression of alpha1 and alpha2/delta1 subunits of L-type high voltage-gated calcium channels after sustained ethanol exposure in cerebral cortical neurons. *J. Pharmacol. Sci.*, 2006, 102, 221-230.

[43] Katsura, M; Mohri, Y; Shuto, K et al. Up-regulation of L-type voltage-dependent calcium channels after long term exposure to nicotine in cerebral cortical neurons. *J. Biol. Chem.*, 2002, 277, 7979-7988.

[44] Nasif, FJ; Hu, XT; White, FJ. Repeated cocaine administration increases voltage-sensitive calcium currents in response to membrane depolarization in medial prefrontal cortex pyramidal neurons. *J. Neurosci*, 2005, 25, 3674-3679.

[45] Hitchcott, PK; Zharkovsky, A; File, SE. Concurrent treatment with verapamil prevents diazepam withdrawal-induced anxiety, in the absence of altered calcium flux in cortical synaptosomes. *Neuropharmacology*, 1992, 31, 55-60.

[46] Rabbani, M; Brown, J; Butterworth, AR; Little, HJ. Dihydropyridine-sensitive calcium channels and barbiturate tolerance and withdrawal. *Pharmacol. Biochem. Behav.*, 1994, 47, 675-680.

[47] Whittington, MA; Lambert, JD; Little, HJ. Increased NMDA receptor and calcium channel activity underlying ethanol withdrawal hyperexcitability. *Alcohol. Alcohol.*, 1995, 30, 105-114.

[48] Anderson, SM; Famous, KR; Sadri-Vakili, G et al. CaMKII: a biochemical bridge linking accumbens dopamine and glutamate systems in cocaine seeking. *Nat. Neurosci.*, 2008, 11, 344-353.

[49] Shibasaki, M; Katsura, M; Kurokawa, K; Torigoe, F; Ohkuma, S. Regional differences of L-type high voltage-gated calcium channel subunit expression in the mouse brain after chronic morphine treatment. *J. Pharmacol. Sci.*, 2007, 105, 177-183.

[50] Hayashida, S; Katsura, M; Torigoe, F; Tsujimura, A; Ohkuma, S. Increased expression of L-type high voltage-gated calcium channel alpha1 and alpha2/delta subunits in mouse brain after chronic nicotine administration. *Brain. Res. Mol. Brain. Res.*, 2005, 135, 280-284.

[51] Shibasaki, M; Kurokawa, K; Ohkuma, S. Upregulation of L-type Ca(v)1 channels in the development of psychological dependence. *Synapse*, 2010, 64, 440-444.

[52] Rajadhyaksha, A; Husson, I; Satpute, SS et al. L-type Ca^{2+} channels mediate adaptation of extracellular signal-regulated kinase 1/2 phosphorylation in the ventral tegmental area after chronic amphetamine treatment. *J. Neurosci.*, 2004, 24, 7464-7476.

[53] Earl, DE; Das, P; Gunning, WT; Alvarez, FJ; Tietz, EI. Ca^{2+}/Calmodulin-Dependent Protein Kinase II Localization and Autophosphorylation within Hippocampal CA1 Excitatory Postsynapses during Flurazepam Withdrawal. *Society for Neuroscience Abstracts*, 2011,

[54] ffrench-Mullen, JM; Barker, JL; Rogawski, MA. Calcium current block by (-)-pentobarbital, phenobarbital, and CHEB but not (+)-pentobarbital in acutely isolated hippocampal CA1 neurons: comparison with effects on GABA-activated Cl- current. *J. Neurosci.*, 1993, 13, 3211-3221.

[55] Yamakage, M; Matsuzaki, T; Tsujiguchi, N; Honma, Y; Namiki, A. Inhibitory effects of diazepam and midazolam on Ca^{2+} and K^+ channels in canine tracheal smooth muscle cells. *Anesthesiology*, 1999, 90, 197-207.

[56] Earl, DE; Tietz, EI. Inhibition of Recombinant L-Type Voltage-Gated Calcium Channels by Positive Allosteric Modulators of GABAA Receptors. *J. Pharmacol. Exp. Ther.*, 2011, 337, 301-311.

[57] Griffiths, RR; Johnson, MW. Relative abuse liability of hypnotic drugs: a conceptual framework and algorithm for differentiating among compounds. *J. Clin. Psychiatry*, 2005, 66 Suppl 9, 31-41.

[58] Zeng, X; Xie, XH; Tietz, EI. Reduction of GABA-mediated inhibitory postsynaptic potentials in hippocampal CA1 pyramidal neurons following oral flurazepam administration. *Neuroscience*, 1995, 66, 87-99.

[59] Zeng, XJ; Tietz, EI. Role of bicarbonate ion in mediating decreased synaptic conductance in benzodiazepine tolerant hippocampal CA1 pyramidal neurons. *Brain Res.*, 2000, 868, 202-214.
[60] Zeng, X; Tietz, EI. Depression of early and late monosynaptic inhibitory postsynaptic potentials in hippocampal CA1 neurons following prolonged benzodiazepine administration: role of a reduction in Cl-driving force. *Synapse*, 1997, 25, 125-136.
[61] Van Sickle, B; Cox, A; Schak, K; John, GL; Tietz, E. Chronic benzodiazepine administration alters hippocampal CA1 neuron excitability: NMDA receptor function and expression(1). *Neuropharmacology*, 2002, 43, 595-606.
[62] Sans, N; Vissel, B; Petralia, RS et al. Aberrant formation of glutamate receptor complexes in hippocampal neurons of mice lacking the GluR2 AMPA receptor subunit. *J. Neurosci.*, 2003, 23, 9367-9373.
[63] Barria, A; Malinow, R. NMDA receptor subunit composition controls synaptic plasticity by regulating binding to CaMKII. *Neuron*, 2005, 48, 289-301.
[64] Nong, Y; Huang, YQ; Salter, MW. NMDA receptors are movin' in. *Curr. Opin. Neurobiol.*, 2004, 14, 353-361.
[65] Groc, L; Heine, M; Cognet, L et al. Differential activity-dependent regulation of the lateral mobilities of AMPA and NMDA receptors. *Nat. Neurosci.*, 2004, 7, 695-696.
[66] Tovar, KR; Westbrook, GL. Mobile NMDA receptors at hippocampal synapses. *Neuron*, 2002, 34, 255-264.
[67] Strack, S; Colbran, RJ. Autophosphorylation-dependent targeting of calcium/ calmodulin-dependent protein kinase II by the NR2B subunit of the N-methyl- D-aspartate receptor. *J. Biol. Chem.*, 1998, 273, 20689-20692.
[68] Strack, S; McNeill, RB; Colbran, RJ. Mechanism and regulation of calcium/calmodulin-dependent protein kinase II targeting to the NR2B subunit of the N-methyl-D-aspartate receptor. *J. Biol. Chem.*, 2000, 275, 23798-23806.
[69] Gardoni, F; Mauceri, D; Fiorentini, C et al. CaMKII-dependent phosphorylation regulates SAP97/NR2A interaction. *J. Biol. Chem.*, 2003, 278, 44745-44752.
[70] Shen, G; Tietz, EI. Down-regulation of synaptic GluN2B subunit-containing N-methyl-D-aspartate receptors: A physiological brake on CA1 Neuron {alpha}-amino-3-hydroxy-5-methyl-4-isoxazolepropionic

acid hyperexcitability during benzodiazepine withdrawal. *J. Pharmacol. Exp. Ther*, 2011, 336, 265-273.

[71] Das, P; Zerda, R; Alvarez, FJ; Tietz, EI. Immunogold electron microscopic evidence of differential regulation of GluN1, GluN2A and GluN2B, NMDA-type glutamate receptor subunits in rat hippocampal CA1 synapses during benzodiazepine withdrawal. *J. Comp. Neurol.*, 2010, 518, 4311-4328.

[72] Erreger, K; Chen, PE; Wyllie, DJ; Traynelis, SF. Glutamate receptor gating. *Crit. Rev. Neurobiol.*, 2004, 16, 187-224.

[73] Sobczyk, A; Scheuss, V; Svoboda, K. NMDA receptor subunit-dependent [Ca^{2+}] signaling in individual hippocampal dendritic spines. *J. Neurosci.*, 2005, 25, 6037-6046.

[74] Bayer, KU; De Koninck, P; Leonard, AS; Hell, JW; Schulman, H. Interaction with the NMDA receptor locks CaMKII in an active conformation. *Nature*, 2001, 411, 801-805.

[75] Bayer, KU; LeBel, E; McDonald, GL; O'Leary, H; Schulman, H; De Koninck, P. Transition from reversible to persistent binding of CaMKII to postsynaptic sites and NR2B. *J. Neurosci.*, 2006, 26, 1164-1174.

[76] Shen, G; Mohamed, MS; Das, P; Tietz, EI. Positive allosteric activation of $GABA_A$ receptors bi-directionally modulates hippocampal glutamate plasticity and behaviour. *Biochem. Soc. Trans.*, 2009, 37, 1394-1398.

[77] Tabakoff, B; Hoffman, PL. Ethanol, sedative hypnotics, and glutamate receptor function in brain and cultured cells. *Behav. Genet.*, 1993, 23, 231-236.

[78] Ulrichsen, J; Bech, B; Ebert, B; Diemer, NH; Allerup, P; Hemmingsen, R. Glutamate and benzodiazepine receptor autoradiography in rat brain after repetition of alcohol dependence. *Psychopharmacology (Berl)*, 1996, 126, 31-41.

[79] Floyd, DW; Jung, KY; McCool, BA. Chronic ethanol ingestion facilitates N-methyl-D-aspartate receptor function and expression in rat lateral/basolateral amygdala neurons. *J. Pharmacol. Exp. Ther.*, 2003, 307, 1020-1029.

[80] Hu, XJ; Ticku, MK. Chronic ethanol treatment upregulates the NMDA receptor function and binding in mammalian cortical neurons. *Brain Res. Mol. Brain Res.*, 1995, 30, 347-356.

[81] Hu, XJ; Follesa, P; Ticku, MK. Chronic ethanol treatment produces a selective upregulation of the NMDA receptor subunit gene expression in mammalian cultured cortical neurons. *Brain Res. Mol. Brain. Res.*, 1996, 36, 211-218.

[82] Nagy, J. The NR2B subtype of NMDA receptor: a potential target for the treatment of alcohol dependence. *Curr. Drug Targets. CNS Neurol. Disord.*, 2004, 3, 169-179.

[83] Qiang, M; Denny, AD; Ticku, MK. Chronic intermittent ethanol treatment selectively alters N-methyl-D-aspartate receptor subunit surface expression in cultured cortical neurons. *Mol. Pharmacol.*, 2007, 72, 95-102.

[84] Hardy, PA; Chen, W; Wilce, PA. Chronic ethanol exposure and withdrawal influence NMDA receptor subunit and splice variant mRNA expression in the rat cerebral cortex. *Brain Res.*, 1999, 819, 33-39.

[85] Lovinger, DM; White, G; Weight, FF. Ethanol inhibits NMDA-activated ion current in hippocampal neurons. *Science*, 1989, 243, 1721-1724.

[86] Daniell, LC. Effect of anesthetic and convulsant barbiturates on N-methyl-D-aspartate receptor-mediated calcium flux in brain membrane vesicles. *Pharmacology*, 1994, 49, 296-307.

[87] Ford, KA; Wolf, ME; Hu, XT. Plasticity of L-type Ca^{2+} channels after cocaine withdrawal. *Synapse*, 2009, 63, 690-697.

[88] Kauer, JA; Malenka, RC. Synaptic plasticity and addiction. *Nat. Rev. Neurosci.*, 2007, 8, 844-858.

[89] Self, DW. Where's the excitement in psychostimulant sensitization? *Neuropsychopharmacology*, 2002, 26, 14-17.

[90] Boudreau, AC; Ferrario, CR; Glucksman, MJ; Wolf, ME. Signaling pathway adaptations and novel protein kinase A substrates related to behavioral sensitization to cocaine. *J. Neurochem.*, 2009, 110, 363-377.

[91] Wolf, ME. Regulation of AMPA receptor trafficking in the nucleus accumbens by dopamine and cocaine. *Neurotox. Res.*, 2010, 18, 393-409.

[92] Carlezon, WAJ; Nestler, EJ. Elevated levels of GluR1 in the midbrain: a trigger for sensitization to drugs of abuse? *Trends. Neurosci.*, 2002, 25, 610-615.

[93] Mameli, M; Bellone, C; Brown, MT; Luscher, C. Cocaine inverts rules for synaptic plasticity of glutamate transmission in the ventral tegmental area. *Nat. Neurosci.*, 2011, 14, 414-416.

[94] Tan, KR; Brown, M; Labouebe, G et al. Neural bases for addictive properties of benzodiazepines. *Nature*, 2010, 463, 769-774.

[95] Kauer, JA; Malenka, RC. LTP: AMPA receptors trading places. *Nat. Neurosci.*, 2006, 9, 593-594.

[96] Kauer, JA. Learning mechanisms in addiction: synaptic plasticity in the ventral tegmental area as a result of exposure to drugs of abuse. *Annu. Rev. Physiol.*, 2004, 66, 447-475.

[97] Faleiro, LJ; Jones, S; Kauer, JA. Rapid synaptic plasticity of glutamatergic synapses on dopamine neurons in the ventral tegmental area in response to acute amphetamine injection. *Neuropsychopharmacology*, 2004, 29, 2115-2125.

[98] Vekovischeva, OY; Zamanillo, D; Echenko, O et al. Morphine-induced dependence and sensitization are altered in mice deficient in AMPA-type glutamate receptor-A subunits. *J. Neurosci.*, 2001, 21, 4451-4459.

[99] Katsura, M; Ohkuma, S. Functional proteins involved in regulation of intracellular $Ca^{(2+)}$ for drug development: chronic nicotine treatment upregulates L-type high voltage-gated calcium channels. *J. Pharmacol. Sci.*, 2005, 97, 344-347.

[100] Griffiths, RR; Weerts, EM. Benzodiazepine self-administration in humans and laboratory animals--implications for problems of long-term use and abuse. *Psychopharmacology (Berl)*, 1997, 134, 1-37.

[101] Das, P; Lilly, SM; Zerda, R; Gunning, WTr; Alvarez, FJ; Tietz, EI. Increased AMPA receptor GluR1 subunit incorporation in rat hippocampal CA1 synapses during benzodiazepine withdrawal. *J. Comp. Neurol.*, 2008, 511, 832-846.

In: Synaptic Plasticity
Editors: G. N. McMahon et al.

ISBN: 978-1-62081-004-0
© 2012 Nova Science Publishers, Inc.

Chapter III

NEURONAL CALCIUM SENSOR-1 AND SYNAPTIC PLASTICITY: ROLE IN NEUROLOGICAL AND NEUROPSYCHIATRIC DISORDERS

David Fleischmann and Jamie L. Weiss
William Paterson University, Department of Biology,
300 Pompton Road, Wayne, New Jersey, US

ABSTRACT

Calcium (Ca^{2+}) signaling is the main process that neurons use to undergo synaptic transmission and is a vital mechanism underlying neural plasticity. Neuronal Ca^{2+} Sensor-1 (NCS-1), also known as Frequenin, is an EF-hand high-affinity Ca^{2+}-sensing protein that is an important signaling regulator of neurotransmission. Synaptic plasticity is the ability of neuronal connections (synapses) to adapt both chemically and physically to physiologically relevant stimuli such as the synaptic changes that are essential to learning and memory (e.g. neurotransmission and synaptic maintenance). When this process of synaptic plasticity is distorted, the consequences can lead to both neurological diseases and neuropsychiatric disorders. NCS-1 is involved in both short- and long-term synaptic plasticity. It is located on axon terminals as well as dendrites, and is a regulator of neuronal outgrowth. NCS-1 has also been shown to interact with or regulate neuronal mediators of synaptic transmission. These include voltage-gated Ca^{2+} channels, TRPC5 channels, D2 dopamine receptors, IP3 receptors, and signaling proteins implicated in Alzheimer's disease, Parkinson's disease, and X-linked mental retardation. NCS-1 is implicated in autism, schizophrenia, bipolar disorder, and neurodegenerative disorders. In this review, we give a detailed summary of the current knowledge of NCS-1's role in synaptic plasticity, and speculate about the mechanisms linking NCS-1 signaling to neurological disease.

INTRODUCTION

If Ca^{2+} signals malfunction, or if the fine balance of Ca^{2+} abundance is disturbed, this can lead to changes in both short- and long- term synaptic plasticity, as well as neuronal death. This then goes on to cause neurological disorders, such as Alzheimer's disease, or other neuropsychiatric and cognitive disorders, such as schizophrenia, mental retardation, and autism [1]. In the mammalian brain, there are post-synaptic contact points, containing neurotransmitter receptors, called dendritic spines. Dendritic spines are bulb like extensions that come off the dendrites, and increase the surface area for synaptic transmission [2-5]. They form synapses in the brain [2], and can change during learning and memory. Neurological disorders, in addition to having altered Ca^{2+} signaling, display changes in dendritic number and morphology [2].

Neuronal Ca^{2+} Sensor-1 (NCS-1), also known as Frequenin, is an EF-hand Ca^{2+}-sensing protein that, by virtue of its interactions with other proteins, appears at the crossroads of many diverse neural signaling pathways (Figure 1). *In vitro* and *in vivo* studies have localized NCS-1 to the vicinity of Ca^{2+} stores and in dendritic spines. Studies have shown that NCS-1 upregulation activates N-type Ca^{2+} channels [6-8], stimulates the synthesis of neurotrophic factors [9], and helps to regulate neuronal outgrowth [10]. The full mechanisms of these interactions, and their physiological implications, are currently not well understood. However, studies have implicated disturbances in synaptic plasticity and NCS-1 mediated Ca^{2+} signaling in dendritic spines as common underlying pathological themes (See Figure 1). Many proteins that interact with NCS-1 (Figure 1) have been found to regulate dendritic spine shape and signaling, and also have been previously linked to neurological disorders [2]. This mechanism improves learning and memory [11], and helps regenerate damaged neurons [10]. While apparently beneficial, this upregulation has also been seen in patients diagnosed with schizophrenia and bipolar disorder [12].

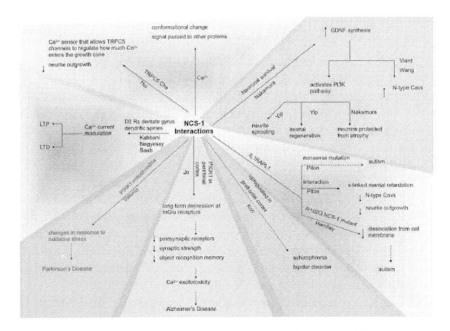

Figure 1. NCS-1 interacts with many other proteins, and is implicated in synaptic plasticity mechanisms affecting both cognitive and neurological disorders. The mechanisms and implications of some interactions are currently not thoroughly understood, but studies have suggested underlying perturbations in synaptic plasticity and NCS-1 mediated Ca^{2+} signaling in dendritic spines. However, NCS-1 can be detected both pre and post- synaptically, having also been show to be present in axon terminals. Many of these binding partners have been found to regulate dendritic spine shape and signaling, and have also been previously linked to neurological disorders. The pathways are color-coded. Orange indicates pre-synaptic, yellow post-synaptic, and pink both pre- and post-synaptic. Pathways in blue are unknown at this time. The surnames listed near the pathways indicate the 1st author of the reference that describes the indicated signaling pathways or how NCS-1 is implicated in a particular disorder.

By contrast, studies have shown that NCS-1 can inhibit voltage-gated Ca^{2+} channels (Cavs) [13]. If dendritic spines become overloaded with inbound Ca^{2+}, enzymes that increase mitochondrial oxidative stress become activated, neuronal outgrowth is reduced, dendritic spines degenerate, and those neurons eventually die [14-17]. These processes are likely to contribute to the development of several types of neurological disorders. NCS-1 may thereby form a functional link between synaptic plasticity, Ca^{2+} current modulation, dopamine signaling, neurological disease, and recovery from physical injury and mitochondrial oxidative stress.

NCS-1 Regulation of Neurotransmission

In healthy neurons, extracellular Ca^{2+} levels far exceed the level of Ca^{2+} in the cytoplasm [18]. Ca^{2+} enters the cell through Cavs, ligand-gated ion channels, and store operated Ca^{2+} channels via the endoplasmic reticulum by inositol 1,4,5-triphosphate receptor activation, or through the mitochondrial uniporter [19]. Synaptic transmission increases intracellular Ca^{2+}, which activates several types of kinases [20]. Intracellular Ca^{2+} levels are partially maintained by Ca^{2+}-binding and Ca^{2+}-buffering proteins, functioning in neuronal Ca^{2+}-signaling pathways [17]. NCS-1 is a Ca^{2+}-binding protein that acts as a Ca^{2+}-signaling sensor that is well placed to regulate neurotransmission. NCS-1 has many interacting proteins and signals in pathways implicated in neurological disorders [13; 21]. Some of these can be categorized as pre- or post- synaptic mechanisms, and some may signal both ways. Figure 1 summarizes and ties these interactions together, as well as links these pathways to disorders of synaptic plasticity and neurology.

NCS-1 is a member of the Calmodulin superfamily of EF-hand Ca^{2+} sensing proteins, NCS subfamily [21]. NCS-1 in mammals is analogous to Frequenin in *Drosophila*. NCS-1 has three functional EF-hand domains, and one inactive domain [21]. NCS-1 binds intracellular Ca^{2+}, undergoes a conformational change that exposes hydrophobic surfaces [22-23], and passes the signal to other proteins, thereby affecting interactions between NCS-1 and signal-receiving proteins, as well as between signal-receiving proteins and other proteins bound to them [24-25]. NCS-1 mediates Cav channels and G-Protein-Coupled-Receptor (GPCR) pathways in neurons and neuroendocrine cells [25-26], in what appears to be pre-synaptic regulation of neurotransmission (Figure 1).

NCS-1 Dendritic Spines and Synaptic Plasticity

Dendritic Spines

Several studies have shown that dendritic spine Ca^{2+} current mediation is important for synaptic plasticity [11; 27]. Dendritic spines are outgrowths from dendrites, consisting of a head and neck, which increase the number of synapses available for neurons to receive input. Early immunolabeling studies in rats showed strong NCS-1 localization to dendrites and dendritic spines [3].

Ca^{2+} enters dendritic spines following excitatory stimulation, but the spine neck hinders its free diffusion [27]. Changes in spine shape shift this compartmentalization, thereby modulating Ca^{2+} current duration [28]. IP_3-mediated Ca^{2+} release from dendritic spines has been shown to initiate Long Term Depression (LTD), a decreased probability of neurotransmitter release, in mice and rats [29]. By contrast, dendritic spines also function in Long Term Potentiation (LTP), an increased probability of neurotransmitter release, through "crosstalk" that enlarges neighboring spines, reduces these neighbors' threshold for potentiation, and increases information storage capacity [30]. Studies in mouse hippocampal pyramidal cells and cultured rat hippocampal slices demonstrated that the decrease in the LTP threshold lasted for 10 minutes, and spread in two directions over a distance of 10 µm. Studies have demonstrated this dendritic spine development depends heavily on continued synaptic stimulation, and helps determine neuronal survival. A loss of afferent input results in a loss of dendritic spines, and their reappearance when innervation is restored [31]. Dendritic spine degeneration in cultured striatal-cortical [16] and hippocampal [15] neurons causes a very large increase in excitatory post-synaptic Ca^{2+} currents, which eventually lead to neuronal cell death by activating Ca^{2+}-dependent enzymes that catabolize cell components and increasing nitric oxide and free radical synthesis [16-17]. Thus, dendritic spine mediation of synaptic plasticity presents a "use it or lose it" phenomenon, with dendritic spine stability being important for neuronal survival. A fine balance is required for the Ca^{2+} signals needed for activity-based neuroprotection versus too much activation. Over activation of neuronal Ca^{2+} signaling pathways can be very dangerous for neurons as it can lead to Ca^{2+}-induced neurotoxicity via oxidative stress that activates apoptotic-signaling pathways [1; 16-17].

Later work suggested that NCS-1 localization in dendritic spines forms a functional link between synaptic plasticity, Ca^{2+} current modulation, dopamine signaling, and neurological disease [2; 4-5; 32-33]. Some proteins (e.g. dopamine D2 receptor signaling, PTEN in PI3 kinase/Akt signaling pathway, metabotropic Glutamate receptors; Figure 1) previously implicated in autism, schizophrenia, and Alzheimer's Disease have also been found to be involved in regulation of dendritic spine morphology, density, connectivity, and maintenance [2]. These same disorders are also associated in various ways with NCS-1, suggesting a possible structural and/or functional connection [4-9; 13]. *In vitro* double immunoelectron labeling experiments revealed that NCS-1 forms a complex with D2 dopamine receptors in the dendrites and spines of cultured monkey and rat striatum, near intracellular Ca^{2+} stores [4] and excitatory glutamatergic synapses [32]. These findings were later confirmed using *in vivo* immunohistochemistry studies of sectioned brains harvested from adult rhesus monkeys [5]. NCS-1 single immunolabeling was observed both pre- and post-synaptically, in dendritic spines, dendrites, and axon terminals, with the most intense immunolabeling in pyramidal neurons. Double immunolabeling showed colocalization of NCS-1 and D2 dopamine receptors pre- and post-synaptically. NCS-1 reduces dopamine-stimulated D2 receptor phosphorylation and internalization, which functions in synaptic plasticity by decreasing neurotransmitter vesicle release [4]. Dendritic spine dopamine signaling, at D1 and D2 receptors, also functions in synaptic plasticity, by evoking LTP or LTD, depending on dopamine concentration [33]. In this regard, NCS-1 appears to have crucial postsynaptic signaling roles (Figure 1).

NCS-1 in Short- and Long- Term Synaptic Plasticity

Synaptic plasticity occurs when synapses modify their electrochemical signaling in response to stimuli. Stimuli can increase the amount of residual Ca^{2+} in the synapse (34), which binds to Ca^{2+}-sensing proteins, and increases the probability of neurotransmitter release [35]. Neurotransmitter release has a fast synchronous phasic phase and a slow asynchronous tonic phase (36). In the synchronous phase, presynaptic Ca^{2+} currents produce a large and fast synaptic response [37]. In the asynchronous phase, after an action potential, residual Ca^{+2} in the axon terminals allows baseline neurotransmitter release [38]. Short-term plasticity and baseline neurotransmitter release are independently regulated [39]. This synaptic enhancement results, through facilitation, augmentation, and post-tetanic potentiation [40]. However, repeated stimulation may eventually deplete the available neurotransmitter vesicles, resulting in synaptic depression [36]. A mechanism for the decrease in neurotransmitter vesicles can occur through a reduction in GPCR auto-receptor desensitization, such as dopamine-stimulated D2 receptor phosphorylation and internalization [4], affecting the regulation of Cavs [26]. Synaptic plasticity functions in learning and memory, and may also have a role in several psychiatric disorders, including autism, schizophrenia, and Alzheimer's disease [41]. Short-term synaptic plasticity is due to an increase in neurotransmission that can be temporary [40]. Long-term synaptic plasticity starts out as a prolonged increase or decrease in neurotransmission by way of increased neurotransmitter release then leads to more stable changes at the post-synaptic neuron via post-synaptic contact-points (dendritic spines) [29-30]. Synaptic plasticity is studied *in vitro* using cell electrophysiological recordings, and *in vivo* using mouse behavioral assays for spatial memory formation and novel object recognition [42].

NCS-1 is thought to mediate short-term synaptic plasticity by enhancing neurotransmission in several ways. One study suggests that NCS-1 allows postsynaptic neurons to fire more readily in response to repeated stimuli, thereby increasing the probability of neurotransmitter vesicle release. Neurotransmitter vesicle release probability was measured in cultured hippocampal cells transfected with NCS-1 [39]. Single-pulse experiments using the non-competitive NMDA (N-Methyl-D-aspartic acid)-receptor antagonist MK-801 were performed. The measurement was repeated under low extracellular Ca^{2+} conditions. In both cases, NCS-1 did not change baseline release probability. Paired pulses resulted in a higher probability of vesicle release. Paired-pulse stimulation resulted in facilitation of the excitatory postsynaptic current that brought the postsynaptic neuron to its voltage threshold. NCS-1 transfection of hippocampal cultures did not change the amplitude of the baseline synaptic response after the first stimulus. Increasing the pulse frequencies resulted in NCS-1 facilitation after the second stimulus and there was no change observed in Ca^{2+} currents or Ca^{2+} channel activation kinetics. In contrast other studies reported P/Q-type Cav current changes by disrupting NCS-1 activity in the Calyx of Held (large auditory nucleus) [43] and also observed in bovine adrenal chromaffin cells [13; 25-26].

Another study has shown that NCS-1 also regulates the Cav currents in neuronal growth cones [8; 13], which are important for outgrowth and branching function in learning and memory [11], and regeneration after injury [9-10]. Neuronal growth occurs only at an optimal intracellular Ca^{2+} level [44]. NCS-1 also appears to act as the Ca^{2+} sensor that allows Transient Receptor Potential Channel 5 (TRPC5) channels to control how much Ca^{2+} enters the growth cone [45]. NCS-1 binding to the C-terminus of TRPC5 decreases neurite outgrowth. In contrast, NCS-1 has been demonstrated to increase neurite outgrowth through upregulation of N-type Ca^{2+} channels [6-7]. These contrasting studies suggest that NCS-1 may be a mediator of neurite outgrowth where it inhibits via TRPC5 channels but enhances via N-type channel activation. Thus, NCS-1 either inhibits or enhances outgrowth and branching, depending on its interacting partners and active signaling pathways [13]. NCS-1 also ensures there is neither too much nor too little neurotransmitter exocytosis, by activating PI4 kinaseIIIβ [13], which leads into the phosphoinositide pathway regulating membrane trafficking. This increases the intracellular concentration of phosphatidylinositol 4,5-bisphosphate (PIP2), which is needed for regulation of neurotransmitter exocytosis [46], and likely allows TRPC5 channels to translocate to neuronal growth cones [47]. TRPC5 incorporation into the cell membrane may also be dependent on Phosphatidylinositol 3-Kinase (PI3K) [47], which is also important for repair and protection of damaged neurons [9-10]. PI3K is also important for activity dependent N-type Cavs insertion into the cell membrane [48]. In contrast, NCS-1 has been shown to mediate long-term synaptic plasticity via LTD metabotropic glutamate receptor (mGluR) signaling in the perirhinal cortex [49]. Therefore, it appears that NCS-1 can both regulate exocytosis, by regulating PIP2 levels and Ca^{2+} channel activity, which in turn regulates both neurotransmission and neurite outgrowth [13]. In this manner, NCS-1 has both pre- and post- synaptic effects on synaptic plasticity [13] (Figure 2).

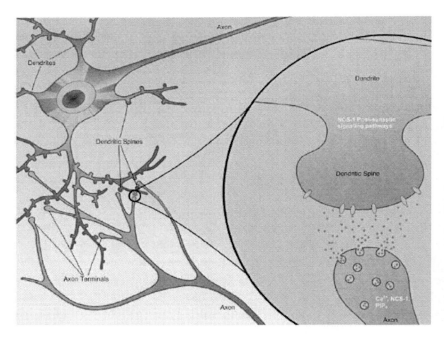

Figure 2. NCS-1 signaling can occur both pre- and post- synaptically. Studies have localized NCS-1 to the vicinity of Ca^{2+} stores, in dendritic spines, indicating post-synaptic local signaling. Dendritic spines are outgrowths from dendrites, consisting of a head and neck, which increase the number of synapses available for neurons to receive input. NCS-1 has also been detected in axon terminals, indicating pre-synaptic localization and signaling.

NCS-1-MEDIATED SYNAPTIC PLASTICITY IN LEARNING AND MEMORY

NCS-1 upregulation has been shown to affect mechanisms of learning and memory in worms and rodents. NCS-1 over expression in *C. elegans* worms resulted in faster conditioned learning of isothermal tracking, and longer retention [50]. In rodents NCS-1 is highly expressed in the hippocampus, in a uniform pattern [51]. Most NCS-1 mRNA was found in dentate gyrus granule cells, with less expression in CA1 and CA3 pyramidal neurons. One study suggests that NCS-1 mRNA induction may be part of the transcriptional response to LTP. LTP was induced at the perforant path dentate granule cell synapse in awake-rats. There was a strong, sustained increase in NCS-1 post-synaptic expression. This occurred at time intervals that correlated with a transition from the LTP early phase to the protein synthesis-dependent late phase [51].

Due to the interaction between NCS-1 and dentate gyrus D2 receptors, NCS-1 overexpression in the adult dentate gyrus (DG) of transgenic mouse strain (DGNCS-1) increased exploration, plasticity, and acquisition of spatial memory [42]. Both DGNCS-1 mice and littermates preferred displaced and novel objects, which indicated no change in spatial learning. After reducing the time for the mice to become familiar with objects and object locations, only the DGNCS-1 mice were able to distinguish between displaced and stationary objects, even after a 24-hour break. The interaction between NCS-1 and the D2 receptor in the dentate gyrus functions in multimodal memory. In DGNCS-1 mice, D2 receptor expression increased at the surface of the dentate gyrus molecular layer, where dopamine influences synaptic plasticity and memory formation. NCS-1 interaction with the D2 receptor was tested using an interfering peptide. The D2 receptor surface levels decreased in dissociated rat hippocampal cultures and mouse hippocampal slices. The DGNCS-1 mice had a lower threshold and higher ceiling for long-term potentiation. In non-fearful environments, the DGNCS-1 mice spent twice as much time rearing as littermate controls, and more time exploring. Direct infusion of the interfering peptide into the dentate gyrus of mice in a non-fearful environment resulted in the same rearing behaviors in both strains, which indicated the NCS-1 interaction with the D2 receptor encourages exploratory rearing. The DGNCS-1 mice also spent twice as much time as littermates searching for a hidden submerged platform in the target quadrant of the Morris water maze, and found it faster. This strongly suggests that the DGNCS-1 mice were better able to learn and remember where the platform was located. When displaced and stationary objects were introduced over a short period of time, only the DGNCS-1 mice were able to distinguish between them. To determine if NCS-1 and the D2 receptor help mediate the rapid acquisition of spatial memory, a higher dose of the interfering peptide was injected into the dentate gyrus. Spatial memory formation was prevented, but novel object recognition, which relies on other brain regions and single-modality memory, was unchanged [42].

NCS-1 SIGNALING IN NEUROLOGICAL DISEASE AND PSYCHIATRIC DISORDERS

NCS-1 Implicated in Mental Impairment

NCS-1 is implicated in X-linked mental retardation through an association with a protein previously demonstrated to decrease Ca^{2+} channel activity and neurite outgrowth. A 150 amino acid extension of IL1RAPL1 (Interleukin-1 Receptor Accessory Protein-Like 1) interacts with NCS-1 [52]. IL1RAPL1 appears to function in down-regulation of N-type Cav channels, Ca^{2+}-dependent exocytosis, and neurite outgrowth [7; 53]. IL1RAPL1 also seems to be involved in synapse formation and transmission during development [54]. It has previously been shown that non-overlapping deletions and a nonsense mutation in IL1RAPL1 cause non-specific X-linked mental retardation [55]. When IL1RAPL1 interacts with NCS-1, N-type Cav channels are inhibited, which decreases neurite outgrowth [52]. In contrast, NCS-1 mediates N-type Cav upregulation in response to neuronal injury, and associated increases in neurite sprouting, through the activation of the anti-apoptotic PI3K/Akt pathway, which increases growth factor synthesis [9].

NCS-1 Implicated in Schizophrenia and Bipolar Disorder

NCS-1 is implicated in schizophrenia and bipolar disorder [56-57]. Schizophrenic and bipolar patients have upregulated NCS-1 in their dorsolateral prefrontal cortex, a brain region involved in working memory and executive functions [12]. Chlorpromazine derivatives, such as thorazine and phenothiazine, exhibit Ca^{2+}-dependent binding to the functional EF-hands of

NCS-1 [58]. These typical antipsychotics antagonize the D2 dopamine receptor with high binding affinity [59]. Given that NCS-1 also binds directly to both the long and short form of the D2 dopamine receptor and that the D2 receptor is a major target for antipsychotic treatment, it appears that NCS-1 signaling is important in schizophrenia and associated disorders. The levels of NCS-1 in white blood cells is also reported to be affected in schizophrenia and bipolar disorder, further linking these two disorders to NCS-1 [60].

NCS-1 Implicated in Autism

NCS-1 may be directly implicated in autism through a mutation that affects its ability to respond appropriately to changing intracellular Ca^{2+} concentrations. A missense mutation in NCS-1, R102Q, has been found in one autistic patient [61]. NMR spectroscopy revealed an exposed surface residue with a high probability of forming a helix. The R102Q mutation affects the structure of the NCS-1 C-terminus, the domain needed to bind to IL1RAPL1. A nonsense mutation in IL1RAPL1, different from that which causes x-linked mental retardation, has been found in one autistic patient without mental retardation [52]. The NCS-1 R102Q mutation has no effect on binding affinity for Ca^{2+} and IL1RAPL1, intercellular colocalization, expression, or inhibitory Ca^{2+} signaling. The mutant R102Q and wild type forms of NCS-1 differ in their response to elevated intracellular Ca^{2+}. Early experiments suggested the existence of multiple NCS-1 pools, due to detergent-sensitive immunostaining [3]. Indeed, it was later discovered that, due to its N-terminal myristoylation [21; 23], wild type NCS-1 binds to the cell membrane when intracellular Ca^{2+} is high [61]. By contrast, NCS-1 R102Q is less able to dissociate from the cell membrane under normal conditions, and so is not affected by increased intracellular Ca^{2+}. The functional mechanism of the resulting aberrant signaling between neurons due to the NCS-1 R102Q mutation, and how it relates to autism, is presently unknown.

NCS-1 Implicated in Alzheimer's Disease

Several *in vitro*, RNA interference, and electrophysiological studies in mice and rats have suggested a possible link between NCS-1 induced LTD, recognition memory deterioration, and Alzheimer's disease. A major symptom of Alzheimer's disease is a loss of recognition memory (62). Recognition memory involves long-term decreased responses to repeated stimuli that be modeled as LTD (63). NCS-1 mediates LTD at metabotropic Glutamate receptors (mGluR), but not at N-Methyl-D-Aspartate (NMDA) receptors. The group 1 metabotropic glutamate receptor agonist DHPG was applied to *in vivo* rat hippocampus [64]. A concentration that can induce synaptic plasticity, as slow onset potentiation, significantly increased NCS-1 expression after 8 and 24 hours. Knocking out NCS-1 using RNA interference stopped mGluR LTD, but not NMDA receptor mediated LTD [63]. Electrophysiological recordings of field excitatory postsynaptic potentials in hippocampal slices from knockout and transgenic mice expressing NCS-1-EGFP have also shown a significant decrease in short term synaptic plasticity [65].

NCS-1 mediates LTD at mGluR receptors in the perirhinal cortex, adjacent to the hippocampus, where it also interacts with a protein known to enhance learning and memory. LTD in the perirhinal cortex is involved in visual object recognition memory [66]. There NCS-1 interacts with the Bin–Amphiphysin–Rvs (BAR) domain of another Ca^{2+}-sensing protein, Protein Interacting With C-Kinase-1 (PICK1), in an unknown but regulated way [63]. PICK1 has been shown to increase the number of postsynaptic membrane receptors in hippocampal neurons, and hence synaptic strength for learning and memory [67]. Perhaps the NCS-1 mediated LTD and interaction with PICK1 interferes with proper membrane trafficking, resulting in fewer postsynaptic receptors, decreased synaptic strength, and loss of object recognition memory. NCS-1 was co-immunoprecipitated with GluR1, GluR2, and PICK1, in perirhinal cortex protein homogenates [63]. Assays using lysates from perirhinal cortices showed stronger interaction between NCS-1 and PICK1 when Ca^{2+} was present. DHPG-treated brain lysates showed stronger NCS-1-PICK1 interaction than in controls. NCS-1 and PICK1 may bind directly in response to elevated Ca^{2+} levels. Since the NCS-1 interaction with PICK1 is stimulated by mGluR receptor activation, but not by NMDA receptor activation, the interaction may be promoted by the activation of Protein Kinase C (PKC) bound to PICK1 [63].

Aberrant intracellular Ca^{2+} signaling may also be involved in Alzheimer's disease. Ca^{2+} indicator dyes have shown a Ca^{2+} overload in dendritic spines [68], and increased Ca^{2+} in the cytoplasm in neurons near amyloid plaques [69]. Soluble neurotoxic Aβ molecules may be released and form a β sheet that creates Ca^{2+} pores [70]. This dendritic spine degeneration allows an abnormally large, over stimulating inbound Ca^{2+} flow, which activates Ca^{2+}-dependent enzymes that catabolize cell components, increases the synthesis of nitric oxide and associated free radicals, and becomes excitotoxic [16-17].

Perhaps this Ca^{2+} influx is involved in the interaction of NCS-1 with PICK1. Abnormal Tau Ca^{2+}-dependent phosphorylation and proteolysis may also occur in Alzheimer's disease [71].

NCS-1 Implicated in Parkinson's Disease

NCS-1 may be implicated in Parkinson's disease through an interaction with proteins known to cause neurodegeneration. A nonsense and a missense mutation have been found in the kinase domain of Phosphatase/TENsin (PTEN) Homology on Chromosome 10- INduced putative Kinase 1 (PINK1), in three consanguineous families known to carry the PARK6 locus [72]. PARK6 gene mutations have previously been linked to an early-onset hereditary form of Parkinson's disease [73]. The PINK1 gene codes for a kinase targeted to the mitochondria, that may help protect cells from neurodegeneration caused by oxidative stress [72]. In zebra fish, loss of PINK1 function increases intracellular levels of caspase-3 and reactive oxygen species, resulting in neurodegeneration [74]. Also in zebra fish, NCS-1 interacts with PINK1, but the nature of the interaction, and how it might contribute to the development of Parkinson's disease, is currently unknown [75].

NCS-1 Implicated in Neuronal Survival and Linked to Neurodegeneration

NCS-1 protects neurons from environmental stress. In the first study to directly point to a curical role for NCS-1 in neuronal survival, NCS-1 and the dominant negative mutant NCS-1 E120Q were overexpressed in primary cultured embryonic rat cortical neurons [9]. NCS-1 E120Q has impaired Ca^{2+} binding, due to a mutation at position 120 of glutamate to glutamine in the third EF hand [25], but normal protein-protein interactions [76]. The change in Ca^{2+} binding NCS-1 E120Q therefore competes with the wild type NCS-1, disrupting the wild type's function. Both cell populations were stressed by B27 withdrawal from the culture medium. Cells overexpressing wild type NCS-1 survived, but cells overexpressing NCS-1 E120Q did not. In cell populations where B27 was kept in the culture medium, cells overexpressing NC-1 E120Q had more cytotoxicity than cells overexpressing wild type NCS-1. PC12 cells were transfected with NCS-1, differentiated into neuron-like cells, and exposed to hydrogen peroxide (H_2O_2). Cells overexpressing NCS-1 sustained insignificant cytotoxicity relative to controls. This suggested that NCS-1 made the PC12 cells more tolerant of hydrogen peroxide [9]. When combined with the previous studies of the NCS-1 interaction with the PINK1 gene [75], these results suggest that NCS-1 may mediate PINK1 neuroprotection from mitochondrial oxidative stress.

NCS-1 also protects neurons from physical stress. One side of the vagus nerve was axotomized in adult rats, and infected with adenoviral vectors encoding NCS-1 wild type, NCS-1 E120Q, and Enhanced Green Fluorescent Protein (EGFP) [9]. There was significant cytotoxicity on the injured side in neurons transfected with NCS-1 E120Q. Unilateral vagal axotomy (nerve trans-section) was performed in adult rats. The brainstems, including the bilateral dorsal motor nucleus of the vagus (DMV) neurons, were isolated, between 1 day and 2 months later. Immunohistochemical staining of frozen sections showed increased NCS-1 expression in the DMV, starting 1 day post-injury, peaking after 1 week, and decreasing over 2 months. Quantitative immunoblot analysis 1 day and 1 week post-injury confirmed these results. NCS-1 expression was also upregulated after continuous treatment with colchicine for 4 days, which interferes with tubulin polymerization and axonal transport [9].

NCS-1 has been shown to protect neurons from stress by increasing neurotrophic factor synthesis, which up-regulates N-type Cav channels, and activates an anti-apoptotic pathway involved in neurite sprouting and regeneration [6]. Neuronal injury increases Glial Cell Line-Derived Neurotrophic Factor (GDNF) synthesis, which activates the Phosphatidylinositol 3-Kinase (PI3K/Akt) pathway [9]. When Akt/PKB is activated by phosphorylation, and bound to substrates PtdIns(3,4)P_2 and PtdIns(3,4,5)P_3, it moves to the plasma membrane. Primary cultured cortical neurons were treated with GDNF for 2 days after B27 withdrawal. Neuronal survival was significantly greater than controls. Cells expressing NCS-1 E120Q did not show an increase in survival after GDNF treatment. Immunoblot analysis showed that NCS-1 expression increased after GDNF administration, due to increased protein synthesis rather than reduced degradation, because GDNF did not increase NCS-1 expression after the protein synthesis inhibitor cycloheximide was administered. In the absence of B27, primary cultured cortical neurons expressing wild type NCS-1 had significantly increased Akt phosphorylation, but those expressing NCS-1 E120Q did not. Wild type NCS-1 overexpression further increased Akt phosphorylation, but NCS-1 E120Q overexpression suppressed it. Cultured cortical neurons were pre-treated with LY294002, which inhibits PI3-K. Neuronal survival induced by GDNF and NCS-1 did not occur. Pre-treatment with PD98059, which inhibits MAPK kinase, did not interfere with this induced neuronal survival. This indicates that NCS-1 mediates neuronal survival through the PI3-K-Akt pathway, not the MAPK pathway, in cultured cortical neurons. The GFP-tagged pleckstrin homology (PH) domain of Akt/PKBα (EGFP-Akt/PKB-PH) was synthesized, and transfected into CCL39 cells, along with NCS-1 or E120Q. CCL39 cells normally have low NCS-1 endogenous expression. NCS-1 overexpression resulted in Akt/PKB-PH localization to the neuron peripheries, whereas E120Q overexpression resulted in diffuse localization. This indicated that NCS-1 increased the levels of PtdIns(3,4)P_2 and PtdIns(3,4,5)P_3, thereby activating Akt/PKB [9].

A more recent study has shown that NCS-1 overexpression through the PI3K/Akt pathway induces collateral neurite sprouting and axonal regeneration. When the PI3K/Akt pathway was blocked in primary cultures of adult mammalian neurons, using the inhibitor LY294002, there were significant decreases in the number of neurites from cell bodies, and the number of sprouts from those neurites [10]. A minimal human immunodeficiency virus-based lentiviral vector, HIV-GFP-NCS-1, was synthesized, expressing NCS-1 and GFP, under the control of cytomegalovirus and spleen focus-forming virus promoters. A control vector was synthesized, HIV-GFP, expressing only GFP, under the control of the cytomegalovirus promoter. Primary adult rat cortical neurons transduced with HIV-GFP-NCS-1 had significant sprouting from both cell bodies and neurites, relative to controls. To determine the types of sprouting neurites, Microtubule-Associated Protein 2 (MAP2) was used to immunolabel dendrites and axons. Increased sprouting was seen on dendrites and axons in neurons transduced with HIV-GFP-NCS-1. HIV-GFP-NCS-1 or control HIV-GFP was injected into the forelimb and hind limb regions of the left sensor motor cortex in adult Wistar rats. Three weeks later, a unilateral pyramidal tract lesion was created, which causes CorticoSpinal Tract (CST) denervation on the other side of the spinal cord. In the cortical spinal neurons overexpressing NCS-1, there was a significant increase in the number of GFP-labeled fibers sprouting across the midline, into the denervated side of the cervical and lumbar spinal cord regions [10].

NCS-1 overexpression through the PI3K/Akt pathway results in significant sensor motor improvement. Sensor motor function was observed for 6 weeks after corticospinal tract denervation. Forelimb extension and grasping were tested using the staircase reaching apparatus [10]. Forelimb and hind limb function were assessed using the grid exploration test. The rats transduced with NCS-1 showed significant sensor motor improvement over controls. Limb misplacement became comparable to rats that received sham transductions. A second lesion was made in the medullar level of the intact pyramidal tract. The sensor motor recovery in the NCS-1 transduced rats was eliminated. CST-denervated limbs in the NCS-1 transduced rats had a larger ElectroMyoGraphic (EMG) response and elbow flexion after 3 pulses of electrical stimulation, relative to controls. Chiseling the intact dorsal corticospinal tract at C4 eliminated the EMG and elbow flexion responses. The EMG responses on the denervated side of the spinal cord had to have originated in pathways crossing from the uninjured side. These results further demonstrated that NCS-1 overexpression had caused sprouting into the CST-denervated side of the spinal cord. NCS-1 overexpression through the PI3K/Akt pathway protects injured corticospinal neurons from atrophy. Adult Wistar rats received lentiviral transductions as before, followed a week later by a pyramidal tract lesion on the same side, at the medullary level [10]. Injecting Fast Blue retrograde tracer into the lesion immediately after its creation identified corticospinal neurons. Control rats had Fast Blue injected into the pyramidal tract at the medullary level, but no lesions or intracortical lentiviral injections. Control GFP-transduced and unlesioned rats exhibited significant cell soma (body) shrinkage. In contrast, the trans-sected corticospinal neurons in NCS-1-transduced rats had no significant cell soma shrinkage [10].

NCS-1 overexpression delayed to post-injury can still induce collateral sprouting and axonal regeneration. Adult Wistar rats received a unilateral pyramidal tract lesion, followed by unilateral intracortical injections of HIV-GFP-NCS-1 or HIV-GFP [10]. NCS-1 transduced rats had a significant increase in the number of GFP-positive collaterals sprouting across the midline into the CST-denervated side, relative to controls. Another group of adult Wistar rats received similar lesions, at the medullary level 2 mm below the decussation, and lentiviral transductions. NCS-1 transduced rats in this cohort had significantly more GFP-positive fibers than controls, and the fibers extended up to 2 mm away from the lesion site. Local sprouting does not exceed 1 mm from the lesion. In this context NCS-1 may enhance neuronal outgrowth but in previous studies with TRPC5 the effect was inhibitory and this effect may depend on the channels and receptor signaling pathways active [13; 45].

NCS-1 Signaling Crosstalk to Neurotrophic Signaling Pathways

The NCS-1 interaction with IL1RAPL1 is likely to cause X-linked mental retardation by downregulating N-type Ca^{2+} channels and decreasing neurite outgrowth [7-8].

In contrast, NCS-1 mediates the newly synthesized growth factors' activation of N-type Cav channels. Under NCS-1 mediation, GDNF activates N-type, but not L-type, Ca^{2+} channels, by increasing the probability they will open [6]. When L-type Cav channels, in cultured *Xenopus* embryo neural tube cells, were blocked with nifedipine, Cav currents were slightly reduced [6]. GDNF administration significantly increased N-type Cav currents. When N-type Cav channels were blocked with omega-conotoxin GVIA, GDNF did not alter Ca^{2+} currents. Cells treated with GDNF exhibited a higher membrane voltage at half-maximal current, relative to controls, with no significant change in channel inactivation. Cav currents were measured in neurons injected with either NCS-1, antisense NCS-1 oligos, or sense NCS-1 oligos, in the presence or absence of GDNF. All neurons treated with GDNF had stronger Ca^{2+} currents, relative to controls. In neurons transfected with antisense NCS-1 oligos, GDNF activation of N-type Ca^{2+} channel currents was reduced [6]. NCS-1-mediated N-type Cav channel activity is likely increased because more channels localize to the cell membrane (26; 48). Rat dorsal root ganglion (DRG) neurons were transfected with GFP-labeled voltage-regulated Ca^{2+} channels. The neurons were exposed to Insulin-Like Growth Factor-1 (IGF-1).

Fluorescence was observed at the cell membrane. Akt/PKB was phosphorylated, which indicated its activation, and the PI3K-induced synthesis of PIP_3. These results demonstrated that increased PIP_3 causes N-type Cav channels to translocate into the cell membrane [48]. NCS-1 acts as a Ca^{2+} sensor that allows TRPC5 channels to control Ca^{2+} influx into the growth cones of developing neurons [45], and the role of PI3K in TRPC5 channel translocation, in the context of enhancing learning and memory. Perhaps a similar mechanism occurs when NCS-1 mediates neurite sprouting and axonal regeneration post injury [10].

CONCLUSION

NCS-1 has been shown to be located in neuronal cell bodies, dendrites and axon terminals. Therefore, NCS-1 can regulate both short- and long- term synaptic plasticity, by controlling neurotransmission at axon terminals and plasticity at dendrites. NCS-1 can also influence postsynaptic signaling, by affecting neurotransmitter receptors and their signaling (Figures 1 and 2). In this way, NCS-1 may mediate the balance between neurotransmission and synaptic plasticity, between neuroprotection and Ca^{2+}-induced neurotoxcity. NCS-1 has been shown to signal via molecules linked to signaling pathways implicated in neurological and neuropsychiatric disorders and there appear to be many avenues for crosstalk [13].

It remains to be seen if NCS-1 has a functional interaction with PINK-1 [75) in mammalian neurons. However, NCS-1's predicted role in mitochondrial oxidative stress fits well with an early study showing that NCS-1 can potentate Nitric Oxide Synthase (NOS), thus being predictive for NCS-1-Ca^{2+} mediated regulation of Nitric Oxide levels [77]. Relatively newer studies linking NCS-1 to PI3K/Akt pathways also link to PINK1, as PTEN is an upstream regulator of PI3K/Akt signaling. These studies implicate NCS-1 in neuronal survival linking NCS-1 to neurodegeneration pathways in Parkinson's disease as the kinase PINK1 is linked to the PI3K/Akt signaling pathway via PTEN [9; 75]. NCS-1 and PTEN have also been linked to the signaling pathways activated in response to chronic stress induced via glucocorticoids in neuropsychiatric disorders. Both NCS-1 and PTEN were shown to be upregulated in mouse cortical neurons after continuous treatment with corticosterone, which is a naturally occurring glucocorticoid, in a recent study [78].

A latest study may link NCS-1's role in autism and dopamine receptor signaling, as the NCS-1 R102Q mutant linked to autism has been reported to have two times higher affinity for the D2 receptor as compared to wild-type NCS-1 [79]. This would be predicted to have an effect on dopamine signaling that could be at least in part contribute to the symptoms of autism [80]. As researchers continue to elucidate NCS-1 signaling mechanisms and the impact of these on the physiology of both neurological and neuropsychiatric disorders, we move closer to more specific and efficient treatments.

In summary, NCS-1 is a mediator of neurotransmission and synaptic plasticity, interacting within signaling pathways important in neuronal survival and synaptic maintenance. If any of these pathways are disrupted, this may lead to cognitive disorders and neurological diseases with neurodegeneration. We look to the future to see if NCS-1 and/or its signaling components will be developed as novel drug targets to treat these disorders.

ACKNOWLEDGMENTS

We thank Karl-Heinz Braunewell for helpful comments and feedback on an earlier version of this manuscript. We also want to thank Chris North for help in creating the figures.

REFERENCES

[1] Braunewell K.H. (2005) The darker side of Ca^{2+} signaling by neuronal Ca^{2+}-sensor proteins: from Alzheimer's disease to cancer. *Trends Pharmacol. Sci.* 26, 345-351.

[2] Penzes P, Cahill ME, Jones KA, VanLeeuwen JE, Woolfrey KM: Dendritic spine pathology in neuropsychiatric disorders. *Nature neuroscience* 14:285-293, 2011.

[3] Martone ME, Edelmann VM, Ellisman MH, Nef P: Cellular and subcellular distribution of the Ca^{2+}-binding protein NCS-1 in the central nervous system of the rat. *Cell and tissue research* 295:395-407, 1999.

[4] Kabbani N, Negyessy L, Lin R, Goldman-Rakic P, Levenson R: Interaction with neuronal Ca^{2+} sensor NCS-1 mediates desensitization of the D2 dopamine receptor. *The Journal of neuroscience* 22:8476, 2002.

[5] Negyessy L, Goldman-Rakic PS: Subcellular localization of the dopamine D2 receptor and coexistence with the Ca^{2+}-binding protein neuronal Ca^{2+} sensor-1 in the primate prefrontal cortex. *The Journal of comparative neurology* 488:464-475, 2005.

[6] Wang CY, Yang F, He X, Chow A, Du J, Russell JT, Lu B: Ca^{2+} binding protein frequenin mediates GDNF-induced potentiation of Ca^{2+} channels and transmitter release. *Neuron* 32:99-112, 2001.

[7] Gambino F, Pavlowsky A, Béglé A, Dupont JL, Bahi N, Courjaret R, Gardette R, Hadjkacem H, Skala H, Poulain B: IL1-receptor accessory protein-like 1 (IL1RAPL1), a protein involved in cognitive functions, regulates N-type Ca^{2+}-channel and neurite elongation. *Proceedings of the National Academy of Sciences* 104:9063, 2007.

[8] Hui K, Feng ZP: NCS-1 differentially regulates growth cone and somata Ca^{2+} channels in Lymnaea neurons. *Eur J Neurosci* 27:631-643, 2008.

[9] Nakamura TY, Jeromin A, Smith G, Kurushima H, Koga H, Nakabeppu Y, Wakabayashi S, Nabekura J: Novel role of neuronal Ca^{2+} sensor-1 as

a survival factor up-regulated in injured neurons. *The Journal of cell biology* 172:1081, 2006.

[10] Yip PK, Wong LF, Sears TA, Yáñez-Muñoz RJ, McMahon SB: Cortical overexpression of neuronal Ca^{2+} sensor-1 induces functional plasticity in spinal cord following unilateral pyramidal tract injury in rat. *PLoS biology* 8:e1000399, 2010.

[11] Jan YN, Jan LY: Dendrites. *Genes. Dev.* 15:2627-2641, 2001.

[12] Koh PO, Undie AS, Kabbani N, Levenson R, Goldman-Rakic PS, Lidow MS: Up-regulation of neuronal Ca^{2+} sensor-1 (NCS-1) in the prefrontal cortex of schizophrenic and bipolar patients. *Proceedings of the National Academy of Sciences* 100:313, 2003.

[13] Weiss J, Hui H, Burgoyne R: Neuronal Ca^{2+} Sensor-1 Regulation of Ca^{2+} Channels, Secretion, and Neuronal Outgrowth. *Cellular and molecular neurobiology* 30:1283-1292, 2010.

[14] Segal M, Greenberger V, Korkotian E: Formation of dendritic spines in cultured striatal neurons depends on excitatory afferent activity. *European Journal of Neuroscience* 17:2573-2585, 2003.

[15] Pilpel Y, Segal M: Activation of PKC induces rapid morphological plasticity in dendrites of hippocampal neurons via Rac and Rho-dependent mechanisms. *European Journal of Neuroscience* 19:3151-3164, 2004.

[16] Segal M: Dendritic spines, synaptic plasticity and neuronal survival: activity shapes dendritic spines to enhance neuronal viability. *European Journal of Neuroscience* 31:2178-2184, 2010.

[17] Marambaud P, Dreses-Werringloer U, Vingtdeux V: Ca^{2+} signaling in neurodegeneration. *Molecular Neurodegeneration* 4, 2009.

[18] Berridge MJ, Lipp P, Bootman MD: The versatility and universality of Ca^{2+} signalling. *Nature Reviews Molecular Cell Biology* 1:11-21, 2000.

[19] Bootman MD, Berridge MJ, Roderick HL: Ca^{2+} signalling: more messengers, more channels, more complexity. *Current biology* 12:R563-R565, 2002.

[20] Berridge MJ, Bootman MD, Roderick HL: Ca^{2+} signaling: dynamics, homeostasis and remodelling. *Nature Reviews Molecular Cell Biology* 4:517-529, 2003.

[21] Burgoyne RD, Weiss JL: The neuronal Ca^{2+} sensor family of Ca^{2+}-binding proteins. *Biochemical Journal* 353:1, 2001.

[22] Cox JA, Durussel I, Comte M, Nef S, Nef P, Lenz SE, Gundelfinger ED: Cation binding and conformational changes in VILIP and NCS-1, two

neuron-specific Ca^{2+}-binding proteins. *Journal of Biological Chemistry* 269:32807, 1994.

[23] Ames JB, Lim S: Molecular structure and target recognition of neuronal Ca^{2+} sensor proteins. *Biochim. Biophys Acta*, Oct 13, 2011, Epub ahead of print.

[24] Weiss J, Burgoyne R: EF-Hand Proteins and Ca^{2+} Sensing: The Neuronal Ca^{2+} Sensors. In *Handbook of Cell Signaling*, Elsevier Science, 2003.

[25] Weiss JL, Archer DA, Burgoyne RD: Neuronal Ca^{2+} sensor-1/frequenin functions in an autocrine pathway regulating Ca^{2+} channels in bovine adrenal chromaffin cells. *Journal of Biological Chemistry* 275:40082, 2000.

[26] Weiss JL, Burgoyne RD: Sense and sensibility in the regulation of voltage-gated $Ca(^{2+})$ channels. *Trends Neurosci.* 25:489-491, 2002

[27] Sabatini BL, Maravall M, Svoboda K: Ca^{2+} signaling in dendritic spines. *Current opinion in neurobiology* 11:349-356, 2001.

[28] Majewska A, Tashiro A, Yuste R: Regulation of spine Ca^{2+} dynamics by rapid spine motility. *The Journal of Neuroscience* 20:8262, 2000.

[29] Miyata M, Finch EA, Khiroug L, Hashimoto K, Hayasaka S, Oda SI, Inouye M, Takagishi Y, Augustine GJ, Kano M: Local Ca^{2+} release in dendritic spines required for long-term synaptic depression. *Neuron* 28:233-244, 2000.

[30] Harvey CD, Svoboda K: Locally dynamic synaptic learning rules in pyramidal neuron dendrites. *Nature* 450:1195-1200, 2007.

[31] Frotscher M, Drakew A, Heimrich B: Role of afferent innervation and neuronal activity in dendritic development and spine maturation of fascia dentata granule cells. *Cerebral Cortex* 10:946, 2000.

[32] Yao W-D, Spealman RD, Zhang J: Dopaminergic signaling in dendritic spines. *Biochemical pharmacology* 75:2055-2069, 2008.

[33] Otani S, Daniel H, Roisin MP, Crepel F: Dopaminergic modulation of long-term synaptic plasticity in rat prefrontal neurons. *Cerebral Cortex* 13:1251, 2003.

[34] Katz B, Miledi R: The role of Ca^{2+} in neuromuscular facilitation. *The Journal of physiology* 195:481, 1968.

[35] Felmy F, Neher E, Schneggenburger R: Probing the intracellular Ca^{2+} sensitivity of transmitter release during synaptic facilitation. *Neuron* 37:801-811, 2003

[36] Catterall WA, Few AP: Ca^{2+} channel regulation and presynaptic plasticity. *Neuron* 59:882-901, 2008.

[37] Llinas R, Steinberg IZ, Walton K: Relationship between presynaptic Ca^{2+} current and postsynaptic potential in squid giant synapse. *Biophysical journal* 33:323-351, 1981.

[38] Atluri PP, Regehr WG: Delayed release of neurotransmitter from cerebellar granule cells. *The Journal of neuroscience* 18:8214, 1998.

[39] Sippy T, Cruz-Martin A, Jeromin A, Schweizer FE: Acute changes in short-term plasticity at synapses with elevated levels of neuronal Ca^{2+} sensor-1. *Nature neuroscience* 6:1031-1038, 2003.

[40] Zucker RS, Regehr WG: Short-term synaptic plasticity. *Annual Review of Physiology* 64:355-405, 2002.

[41] Citri A, Malenka RC: Synaptic plasticity: multiple forms, functions, and mechanisms. *Neuropsychopharmacology* 33:18-41, 2008.

[42] Saab BJ, Georgiou J, Nath A, Lee FJS, Wang M, Michalon A, Liu F, Mansuy IM, Roder JC: NCS-1 in the dentate gyrus promotes exploration, synaptic plasticity, and rapid acquisition of spatial memory. *Neuron* 63:643-656, 2009.

[43] Tsujimoto T, Jeromin A, Saitoh N, Roder JC, Takahashi T: Neuronal Ca^{2+} sensor 1 and activity-dependent facilitation of P/Q-type Ca^{2+} currents at presynaptic nerve terminals. *Science* 295:2276, 2002.

[44] Fields RD, Guthrie PB, Russell JT, Kater SB, Malhotra BS, Nelson PG: Accommodation of mouse DRG growth cones to electrically induced collapse: Kinetic analysis of Ca^{2+} transients and set-point theory. *Journal of neurobiology* 24:1080-1098, 1993.

[45] Hui H, McHugh D, Hannan M, Zeng F, Xu SZ, Khan SH, Levenson R, Beech DJ, Weiss JL: Ca^{2+} sensing mechanism in TRPC5 channels contributing to retardation of neurite outgrowth. *The Journal of physiology* 572:165-172, 2006.

[46] Martin TFJ: PI (4, 5) P2 regulation of surface membrane traffic. *Current opinion in cell biology* 13:493-499, 2001.

[47] Bezzerides VJ, Ramsey IS, Kotecha S, Greka A, Clapham DE: Rapid vesicular translocation and insertion of TRP channels. *Nature cell biology* 6:709-720, 2004.

[48] Viard P, Butcher AJ, Halet G, Davies A, Nurnberg B, Heblich F, Dolphin AC: PI3K promotes voltage-dependent Ca^{2+} channel trafficking to the plasma membrane. *Nature neuroscience* 7:939-946, 2004.

[49] Jo J, Heon S, Kim MJ, Son GH, Park Y, Henley JM, Weiss JL, Sheng M, Collingridge GL, Cho K: Metabotropic glutamate receptor-mediated LTD involves two interacting Ca^{2+} sensors, NCS-1 and PICK1. *Neuron* 60:1095-1111, 2008.

[50] Gomez M, De Castro E, Guarin E, Sasakura H, Kuhara A, Mori I, Bartfai T, Bargmann CI, Nef P: Ca^{2+} signaling via the neuronal Ca^{2+} sensor-1 regulates associative learning and memory in C. elegans. *Neuron* 30:241-248, 2001.

[51] Genin A, Davis S, Meziane H, Doyere V, Jeromin A, Roder J, Mallet J, Laroche S: Regulated expression of the neuronal Ca^{2+} sensor-1 gene during long-term potentiation in the dentate gyrus in vivo. *Neuroscience* 106:571-577, 2001.

[52] Piton A, Michaud JL, Peng H, Aradhya S, Gauthier J, Mottron L, Champagne N, Lafrenire RG, Hamdan FF, Joober R: Mutations in the Ca^{2+}-related gene IL1RAPL1 are associated with autism. *Human molecular genetics* 17:3965, 2008.

[53] Gambino F, Kneib M, Pavlowsky A, Skala H, Heitz Sp, Vitale N, Poulain B, Khelfaoui M, Chelly J, Billuart P, Humeau Y: IL1RAPL1 controls inhibitory networks during cerebellar development in mice. *European Journal of Neuroscience* 30:1476-1486, 2009.

[54] Yoshida T, Mishina M: Zebrafish orthologue of mental retardation protein IL1RAPL1 regulates presynaptic differentiation. *Molecular and Cellular Neuroscience* 39:218-228, 2008.

[55] Bahi N, Friocourt G, Carrie, A, Graham ME, Weiss JL, Chafey P, Fauchereau F, Burgoyne RD, Chelly J: IL1 receptor accessory protein like, a protein involved in X-linked mental retardation, interacts with Neuronal Ca^{2+} Sensor-1 and regulates exocytosis. *Human molecular genetics* 12:1415, 2003.

[56] Bai J, He F, Novikova SI, Undie AS, Dracheva S, Haroutunian V, Lidow MS: Abnormalities in the dopamine system in schizophrenia may lie in altered levels of dopamine receptor-interacting proteins. *Biol. Psychiatry* 56:427-440, 2004.

[57] Kabbani N, Woll MP, Nordman JC, Levenson R: Dopamine Receptor Interacting Proteins: Targeting Neuronal Ca^{2+} Sensor-1/D2 Dopamine Receptor Interaction for Antipsychotic Drug Development. *Curr. Drug Targets*, 2011.

[58] Muralidhar D, Kunjachen Jobby M, Jeromin A, Roder J, Thomas F, Sharma Y: Ca^{2+} and chlorpromazine binding to the EF-hand peptides of neuronal Ca^{2+} sensor-1. *Peptides* 25:909-917, 2004.

[59] Dean B, Scarr E: Antipsychotic drugs: evolving mechanisms of action with improved therapeutic benefits. *Current Drug Targets-CNS and# 38; Neurological Disorders* 3:217-226, 2004.

[60] Torres KC, Souza BR, Miranda DM, Sampaio AM, Nicolato R, Neves FS, Barros AG, Dutra WO, Gollob KJ, Correa H, Romano-Silva MA: Expression of neuronal Ca^{2+} sensor-1 (NCS-1) is decreased in leukocytes of schizophrenia and bipolar disorder patients. *Prog. Neuropsychopharmacol. Biol. Psychiatry* 33:229-234, 2009.

[61] Handley MTW, Lian LY, Haynes LP, Burgoyne RD: Structural and functional deficits in a Neuronal Ca^{2+} Sensor-1 mutant identified in a case of Autistic Spectrum Disorder. *PLoS One* 5:e10534, 2010.

[62] Barbeau E, Didic M, Tramoni E, Felician O, Joubert S, Sontheimer A, Ceccaldi M, Poncet M: Evaluation of visual recognition memory in MCI patients. *Neurology* 62:1317, 2004.

[63] Jo J, Heon S, Kim MJ, Son GH, Park Y, Henley JM, Weiss JL, Sheng M, Collingridge GL, Cho K: Metabotropic glutamate receptor-mediated LTD involves two interacting $Ca(^{2+})$ sensors, NCS-1 and PICK1. *Neuron* 60:1095-1111, 2008.

[64] Brackmann M, Zhao C, Kuhl D, Manahan-Vaughan D, Braunewell KH: MGluRs regulate the expression of neuronal Ca^{2+} sensor proteins NCS-1 and VILIP-1 and the immediate early gene arg3.1/arc in the hippocampus in vivo. *Biochem. Biophys. Res. Commun.* 322:1073-1079, 2004.

[65] Hermainski J, Stockebrand M, Pongs O: Synaptic Plasticity in NCS-1 Knock-Out and NCS-1-EGFP Overexpressing Mice. European Calcium Society Workshop, Smolenice, Slovakia, June 2009.

[66] Barker GRI, Bashir ZI, Brown MW, Warburton EC: A temporally distinct role for group I and group II metabotropic glutamate receptors in object recognition memory. *Learning and Memory* 13:178, 2006.

[67] Hanley JG, Henley JM: PICK1 is a Ca^{2+}-sensor for NMDA-induced AMPA receptor trafficking. *The EMBO journal* 24:3266-3278, 2005.

[68] Kuchibhotla KV, Goldman ST, Lattarulo CR, Wu HY, Hyman BT, Bacskai BJ: A [beta] Plaques Lead to Aberrant Regulation of Ca^{2+} Homeostasis In Vivo Resulting in Structural and Functional Disruption of Neuronal Networks. *Neuron* 59:214-225, 2008.

[69] Busche MA, Eichhoff G, Adelsberger H, Abramowski D, Wiederhold KH, Haass C, Staufenbiel M, Konnerth A, Garaschuk O: Clusters of hyperactive neurons near amyloid plaques in a mouse model of Alzheimer's disease. *Science* 321:1686, 2008.

[70] Mirzabekov TA, Lin M, Kagan BL: Pore formation by the cytotoxic islet amyloid peptide amylin. *Journal of Biological Chemistry* 271:1988, 1996.

[71] Sato S, Xu J, Okuyama S, Martinez LB, Walsh SM, Jacobsen MT, Swan RJ, Schlautman JD, Ciborowski P, Ikezu T: Spatial learning impairment, enhanced CDK5/p35 activity, and downregulation of NMDA receptor expression in transgenic mice expressing tau-tubulin kinase 1. *The Journal of Neuroscience* 28:14511, 2008.

[72] Valente EM, Abou-Sleiman PM, Caputo V, Muqit MMK, Harvey K, Gispert S, Ali Z, Del Turco D, Bentivoglio AR, Healy DG: Hereditary early-onset Parkinson's disease caused by mutations in PINK1. *Science* 304:1158, 2004.

[73] Lücking CB, Dürr A, Bonifati V, Vaughan J, De Michele G, Gasser T, Harhangi BS, Meco G, Denèfle P, Wood NW, Agid Y, Brice A: Association between early-onset Parkinson's disease and mutations in the parkin gene; New England Journal of Medicine 342:1560-1567, 2000

[74] Anichtchik O, Diekmann H, Fleming A, Roach A, Goldsmith P, Rubinsztein DC: Loss of PINK1 function affects development and results in neurodegeneration in zebrafish. *The Journal of Neuroscience* 28:8199, 2008.

[75] Petko JA, Kabbani N, Frey C, Woll M, Hickey K, Craig M, Canfield VA, Levenson R: Proteomic and functional analysis of NCS-1 binding proteins reveals novel signaling pathways required for inner ear development in zebrafish. *BMC Neurosci* 10:27, 2009.

[76] McFerran BW, Weiss JL, Burgoyne RD: Neuronal Ca($^{2+}$) sensor 1. Characterization of the myristoylated protein, its cellular effects in permeabilized adrenal chromaffin cells, Ca($^{2+}$)-independent membrane association, and interaction with binding proteins, suggesting a role in rapid Ca($^{2+}$) signal transduction. *J. Biol. Chem.* 274:30258-30265, 1999.

[77] Schaad NC, De Castro E, Nef S, Hegi S, Hinrichsen R, Martone ME, Ellisman MH, Sikkink R, Rusnak F, Sygush J, Nef P: Direct modulation of calmodulin targets by the neuronal calcium sensor NCS-1. *Proc. Natl. Acad. Sci. USA* 93:9253-9258, 1996.

[78] Howell KR, Kutiyanawalla A, Pillai A (2011) Long-term continuous corticosterone treatment decreases VEGF receptor-2 expression in frontal cortex. PLoS One 6: e20198. 79. Lian LY, Pandalaneni SR, Patel P, McCue HV, Haynes LP, Burgoyne RD: Characterisation of the interaction of the C-terminus of the dopamine D2 receptor with neuronal calcium sensor-1. *PLoS One* 6:e27779, 2011.

[79] Arias-Carrion O, Poppel E: Dopamine, learning, and reward-seeking behavior. *Acta Neurobiol. Exp.* (Wars) 67:481-488, 2007.

In: Synaptic Plasticity
Editors: G. N. McMahon et al.

ISBN: 978-1-62081-004-0
© 2012 Nova Science Publishers, Inc.

Chapter IV

FAULTY PLASTICITY: A COMMON THREAD CONNECTING NEUROLOGICAL DISEASES

*Daniel Montoya**, *Ashley Bofill, and Stephen Gill*
Fayetteville State University, Fayetteville, NC, US

ABSTRACT

Plastic processes, in particular Long Term Potentiation (LTP) and Long Term Depression (LTD), seem to play a role in the development of certain neurological disorders. Both physiological processes are defined by long lasting changes in synaptic transmission and are commonly studied in the hippocampus, although there is evidence of their occurrence in some other brain areas, particularly cortico-striatal networks. It is well known that plasticity is affected in Alzheimer's disease due to a deficiency in N-Methyl-D-Asparte (NMDA) receptors, one of the central elements on which the induction of LTP hinges. The present chapter focuses, however, on recent developments in animal and human studies that associate LTP to other conditions such as Huntington's, Parkinson's, and dystonia. In most cases, plasticity, as indexed by LTP or LTD manipulations, is impaired. In some instances, NMDA receptors are involved together with other neurotransmitters systems. We point out that a unified view of the role of plasticity in disease has not been developed. However, recent models of homeostatic

---

* Corresponding Author:Biopsychology Laboratory. Department of Psychology. Fayetteville State University. Fayetteville, NC 28301. USA. E-mail: dmontoya@uncfsu.edu.

plasticity (a negative feedback mechanism, present in neural populations, that offset excessive excitation or inhibition by adjusting the limits of synaptic strength) may be useful to understand and predict some of the observed effects. We argue that future research has to establish plasticity's contribution, either as a promoter of a given disorder or as a side-effect resulting from other physiological processes.

Keywords: Long Term Potentiation; Homeostatic Plasticity; Humans; Alzheimer's, Parkinson's, Huntington's, dystonia

INTRODUCTION - LONG TERM POTENTIATION AS AN INDEX OF NEURAL PLASTICITY

When looking for physiological candidates to sustain learning and memory, Long Term Potentiation (LTP) is considered one of the most important physiological mechanism studied so far. LTP is a long lasting enhancement in synaptic communication that was originally observed after applying high frequency stimulation to neighboring cells [1]. In their seminal experiments, Bliss and LØmo showed a modification that developed after a train of high frequency stimulation (HFS) was delivered to the perforanth path in the hippocampus. Immediately after this tetanization, an increase in the size of the excitatory postsynaptic potential (EPSP) was recorded in the dentate gyrus. The synaptic changes that they described lasted from 30 minutes to several hours. At that time, synaptic changes that persisted for more than a few milliseconds were unknown. Inadvertently, their work gave credibility to a hypothesis put forward by Donald Hebb in 1949: *"When an axon of cell A is near enough to excite cell B and repeatedly or persistently takes part in firing it, some growth process or metabolic change takes place in one or both cells such that A's efficiency, as one of the cells firing B, is increased"* [2].

Decades of studies established that several different neural pathways in the brain support LTP [3]. In addition, as predicted by Hebbian plasticity, the phenomenon displays very interesting properties, which turns it into a convenient neural correlate of memory [4]. A summary list of LTP properties includes long duration as its main characteristic [5], but also the capacity of producing potentiation only in the stimulated neural paths, a characteristic known as input specificity [6]. Furthermore, a weak stimulation produces LTP only when associated to a strong stimulation, a property identified as associativity or cooperativity [7]. After the induction of LTP, the response can be brought back to basal levels by a train of low frequency stimulation on the same previously potentiated pathway, in a phenomenon known as "depotentiation" [8]. At a neurotransmitter level, the glutamate receptor N-Methyl-D-Aspartate (NMDA) plays a central role in LTP. By an increase in presynaptic glutamate release paired with the delivery of high frequency stimulation, the magnesium blockade at the NMDA receptor is removed, increasing calcium flow into the cell [9]. More recently, it has been established that LTP presents multiple phases based on their persistence over time: LTP1, LTP2 and LTP3 [10]. Each one of these phases is sustained by different molecular and physiological mechanisms. With repeated use of a given pathway and stabilization, LTP produces changes in spine morphology [11], a necessary step for establishing the relationship between physiological changes and learning in vertebrates [12].

A physiological counterpart of LTP has been described under the guise of Long Term Depression (LTD), defined as a decrease in synaptic efficacy after the delivery of long trains (~ 900 pulses) of electrical stimulation administered at a very low frequency (~ 1-10 Hz) [13]. Both processes differ in the protocols used to produce them, but they share some of the basic mechanisms. For example, both are $Ca+2$-dependent phenomena, as well as reliant on NMDAr and protein phosphatases activation [14]. Other studies indicate a crucial role for caspases (specifically caspase-3) in the induction of NMDAr-dependent LTD, a protease usually involved in apoptosis [15]. Early on, much of the research in LTD mechanisms was carried out in slices of very young animals and there was some doubt about the event being present in the adult brain [16]. However, recent evidence shows that it is possible to initiate LTD in older animals (10-14 months old mice) although the evidence does not support a role for NMDAr [17].

Both forms of synaptic activity (LTP and LTD) represent the brain's capacity to sustain plastic changes. Although, it is not clear how neural transmission is connected with thoughts, perceptions and observed behaviors, these mechanisms are a useful window to study the modulatory effects of experience.

LTP IN THE HUMAN CORTEX: RECENT EVIDENCE FROM NON-INVASIVE TECHNIQUES

The phenomenon has been studied extensively at the cellular level in laboratory animals but has not been directly demonstrated in the intact human brain [10], although its presence has been documented using tissue obtained from surgical patients [18, 19]. Using evoked related potentials (ERP), a non-invasive technique that quantifies the brain's electrical response following a stimulus presentation, Teyler and collaborators [20] demonstrated LTP in the human visual cortex. These results were confirmed using functional magnetic resonance [21], which showed an increase in extrastriate visual cortex activity after tetanization with a checkerboard stimulus. A subsequent study of the LTP-like properties in the human cortex demonstrated selective potentiation of orientation-tuned neurons after rapid visual stimulation, a corroboration of specificity [22]. In addition, LTP has also been described in the human auditory cortex utilizing high frequency presentation of auditory pips through the participant's ears [21]. Other lines of evidence confirmed that this phenomenon in humans is NMDAr dependent and confirmed its absence in patients diagnosed with Alzheimer's disease (AD) [23]. While the events illustrated in these studies seem to preserve some of LTP properties, namely, rapid induction and maintenance of a synaptic communication increase for at least an hour, no other property has been systematically tested in the human cortex. For a recent review see [24].

Of special consideration in our endeavor is a form of LTP described in the basal ganglia. The basal ganglia, a set of subcortical nuclei important for the processing of motivation, motor planning and procedural learning [25], receives input predominantly through the striatum [26]. The striatum in itself seems to be in charge of planning and executing motor programs [27], depending on dopaminergic and glutamatergic connections from the cortex [28].

PLASTICITY AND DISEASE PROCESSES

In thinking about the general ways that plastic processes can be affected by disease, stress comes up as one of the first candidates. Since the hippocampus possesses the highest concentration of corticosterone receptors, high levels of corticoids would impact negatively any behavioral function that is dependent on this structure, like memory [3]. As expected, LTP is inhibited by high concentrations of glucocorticoids, while the opposite is true when glucocorticoid levels are low [29-31]. However, it is not always easy to trace a connection between stress and synaptic failure, specially when synaptic or genetic mechanisms may also influence the onset of the disease process.

In this sense, the relationship between plasticity and disease processes has become more compelling since several reports indicate that plasticity is altered in Parkinson's and Huntington's disease as well as some other disorders (see figure 1). Some authors suggest that neurodegenerative processes may be responsible for converting LTD into LTP or vice versa, bringing the system to extreme levels of excitability and instability [32].

We cannot, however, discard other mechanisms that may include NMDAr function abnormality, as described in relationship to Alzheimer's Disease [23]; dopaminergic function deficiency [33]; reduced availability of neurotrophic factors [34] and, especially, cortical and brainstem plasticity deficits [35]. In the following sections we describe the interrelation between plastic processes, like LTP and LTD, and the different ways in which they are affected in neurological diseases. Moreover, a plethora of recent studies indicate that peripheral nerve injuries can initiate a cascade of effects producing plastic changes not only in the spinal cord, but also affecting the brainstem, the thalamus and the cortex [36].

PLASTICITY IN ALZHEIMER'S DISEASE

Alzheimer's disease is the sixth leading cause of deaths in the United States and the fifth leading cause of death in Americans over 65 years of age [37]. AD is the most common type of dementia characterized by a progressive decay of cognitive and functional abilities. It has been proposed that Alzheimer's Disease is the result of synaptic failure [38].

These synaptic changes would show in mild cognitive impairment expressed as an inability, in the beginning, to codify new information, progressing eventually into a full-blown deficiency in declarative memory and, later on, implicit memory. Of particular importance in the pathogenesis of AD seems to be the elevation of the long form of the peptide Aβ42, which aggregates forming plaques in AD patient's brains [39]. Moreover, the β-amyloid is known to inhibit the development of in vivo LTP [40, 41], an effect that can be reversed by the activation of β2 adrenoceptors, but not of β1 adrenoceptors in the dentate gyrus of adult animals [42].

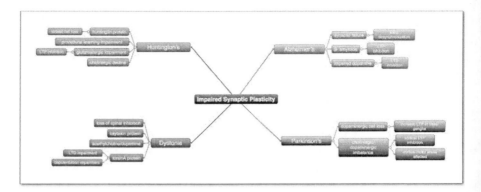

Figure 1. Overview of synaptic plasticity involvement in diseases beyond Alzheimer's disease. The figure highlights the common presence of synaptic alterations and names some of the cellular mechanisms described so far in the literature. The mechanism of impairment is different in each disease process, however, in each case it results in the impairment of synaptic plasticity by affecting the expression of LTP and LTD.

Similarly, other studies show that chronic nicotine treatment prevents Aβ-induced inhibition of basal synaptic transmission and LTP in hippocampal CA1 area [43]. Physiologically, Alzheimer's patients show EEG desynchronization between different cortical areas, especially in the frontal cortex [44].

Evidence also indicates that LTD is impaired in AD patients, which is associated with a dysfunctional dopaminergic transmission [45] together with increased calcium dysregulation [46]. Parallel to this, it has been reported that Alzheimer's patients show an impairment in NMDA receptor function and, subsequently, lack of LTP [23]. All these data point to an intrinsic association between physiological mechanisms of LTP and synaptic failure in Alzheimer's Disease. This synaptic failure, as expected, is highly correlated with, and predicts, the progressive memory decline during the late phase of the disease, disrupting not only memory function but also leading to striking changes in mood and personality.

PLASTICITY IN HUNTINGTON'S DISEASE

Huntington's disease (HD) is a neurodegenerative disorder characterized by progressive motor and cognitive impairments. In the majority of cases, the onset occurs around 35-50 years of age accompanied by a fatal prognosis over the next 15-20 years. Huntington's is characterized by cell loss in the striatum and cortex and the presence of depositions of huntingtin protein, found in aggregates in the cell nucleus [47]. Not surprisingly, humans suffering Huntington's demonstrate impairment in procedural learning [25].

The R6/2 mouse became a very valuable model of Huntington's disease. Using this model it has been possible to pinpoint the convergence of anatomical and chemical elements accompanying the disease, starting with the loss of medium spiny neurons in the striatum [48], which happens along alterations in dopaminergic [49] and glutamatergic transmission [50] - see figure 2. However, the R6/2 model also predicts that progressive cholinergic function decline come before observable symptoms and neural death occurs [51]. These mice show normal hippocampal-dependent memory but they also display difficulty acquiring striatum-dependent memory skills [52].

Animal models developed in the 90's provided a picture of plasticity in the striatum, which seemed to contradict results previously obtained in the hippocampus [53]. Both LTP and LTD were reported with the delivery of high frequency stimulation, which seemed to be dependent on NMDA receptor levels of activation [54]. Facilitation provided by NMDA receptor activation, by removing Mg2 blocking, HFS stimulation produced LTP. Simultaneously, the same kind of stimulation induced LTD under physiological conditions. However, recent studies indicate that cortico-striatal plasticity in rats behaves in the same frequency-dependent manner expected in other areas, with HFS inducing LTP and low frequency stimulation (LFS) inducing in LTD [55].

Additionally, other studies indicate that dopaminergic plasticity is impaired in R6/2's striatal neurons [33]. In the wild type, HFS induce LTP that was successfully blocked by the NMDA antagonist D(-)-2-amino-5-phosphonopentanoic acid (D-AP5) and the D1 receptor antagonist SCH-23390. In adult R6/2 animals LTP was impaired, while at the same time, LFS induced LTD that was not different from the wild type.

There is also evidence that a glutamatergic alteration may play a role: HD patients show an early loss of neurons expressing high levels of NMDAr [56] a process that can be mimicked by the injection of NMDAr agonists such as quinolinic acid (QA) [57] or kainic acid in the striatum [58], with the subsequent loss of striatal projections medium-sized spiny neurons. In addition, a metabolic alteration of a mitochondrial complex II (succinate dehydrogenase, SD) is present in HD. Chronic treatment with an irreversible SD inhibitor, 3-nitropropionic acid (3-NP), can reproduce the motor abnormalities in animal models and, at the same time, is able to induce LTP of corticostriatal synaptic transmission through NMDA glutamate receptors [59]. Applying the same model, Picconi et al [60] described depotentiation of the spiny neurons and an impairment of LTP in cholinergic neurons injecting mitochondrial toxin 3-nitropropionic acid (3-NP) in rats, disturbances that were also present in R6/2 neurons.

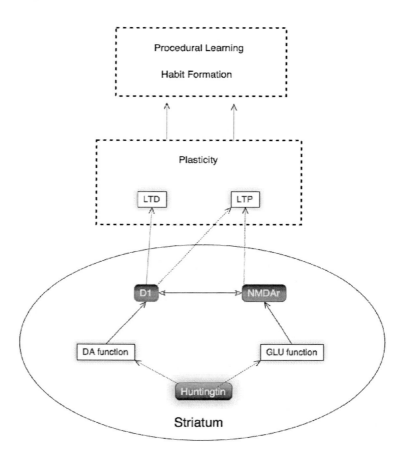

Figure 2. Role of dopaminergic and glutamatergic receptors on striatal plasticity. Huntingtin protein deposits may interfere with D1 receptors and NMDA receptors' activity, which, in turn, produces impairment on plasticity leading to the observed behavioral deficits in HD patients. Based on Kung et al (2007).

Studies in humans have revealed LTP-like changes in the motor cortex by the utilization of paired associative stimulation (PAS), a combination of repetitive electric stimulation of the median nerve followed by transcranial magnetic stimulation (TMS) of the contralateral motor cortex [61]. Using this stimulation paradigm, Crupi and colleagues [35] studied plasticity in

Huntington's patients. The results showed a decrement of potentiation in Huntington's patient similar to the impairment observed in animal models, which indicates that physiological correlates accompany the memory deficits observed in these patients. Clearly, more studies carried out in humans are necessary to determine the reach and characteristics of this phenomenon.

PLASTICITY IN PARKINSON'S DISEASE

Degeneration of dopaminergic neurons in the nigrostriatal pathway is the salient feature of Parkinson's Disease (PD), a disorder accompanied by bradykinesia, tremor and rigidity, initially present in the upper extremities. The cause of this dopaminergic loss is unknown [62], although is present in a predominantly right-handed male population [63]. More recently, some risk factors, like the consumption of fatty acids [64] and several genes [65], have been identified. Other features of PD include speech disfluency [66]; stereotypical walking patterns [67]; impairment in visual memory, visuospatial functions, and naming and calculation [68]; although executive function does not seem to be altered [69]. Two distinctive phases have been established for the development of PD: a pre-clinical phase, which marks the beginning of the physiological disturbances with no evident motor signs, and a clinical phase, characterized by an onset of motor signs and symptoms. The rest of the clinical phase is dominated by the need to manage the progressive symptomatology presented by the disease [63].

A common animal model deployed to study PD is the use of the catecholamine-specific neurotoxin 6-hydroxydopamine (6-OHDA) injected into the substantia nigra, which produces a permanent loss of dopaminergic neurons in the striatum [70, 71]. The lesion resembles the motor impairment, hypokinesia and sensorimotor distress described in PD [72]. Some neurocomputational and neurochemical explanations have been proposed to account for the effect of dopaminergic neurons. According to some neurocomputational models, the loss of dopaminergic neurons increases activity in general leading to a magnification of LTP in the indirect pathway of the basal ganglia [73], while other models focus on an imbalance between acetylcholine and dopamine in the cortex and the striatum [32]. While dopaminergic loss means an increase in acetylcholine activity, the opposite is true for the cortex. The most important element, however, is that chronic dopamine denervation blocks cortico-striatal LTP in animal models, which suggests a role for plasticity, or lack thereof, in the process leading to the disease [74].

As predicted by these observations, Parkinson's Disease patients do not exhibit dopaminergic plasticity. Using the interventional paired associative stimulation (IPAS), a technique that combines electrical stimulation of the right median nerve followed by magnetic stimulation over the left primary motor cortex (M1), Ueki et al [75] were able to clarify the role of basal-ganglia-thalamocortical transmission in PD patients. The technique produces an LTP-like increase in motor evoked potentials when recorded from the muscle output. Despite the fact that the study was carried out with few participants, an increase in evoked potentials was observed only in matched healthy controls but not in the PD patients. More recently, Suppa et al [76] relied on intermittent theta-burst stimulation (iTBS) to induce non-invasive LTP in the motor cortex in Parkinson patients under different dopaminergic medications and -L-Dopa treatment. Following iTBS, the motor evoked potentials in control subjects significantly increased. However, it remained without changes in Parkinson's patients.

PLASTICITY IN DYSTONIA

Long lasting muscle contraction causing automatic movements and abnormal postures in different body parts define dystonia [77]. The disorder can manifest in a generalized form, when several body parts are affected, or in a focalized form, when there is only one body part disturbed by the dystonic movement [78]. In several cases of focal dystonia, the disorder is only manifested when the patient tries to perform a specific movement. Accordingly, varying forms of focal dystonia received names based on the kind of movement affected: writer's cramp, pianist's cramp, and typist's cramp, are all examples of occupational dystonias. Transcranial magnetic stimulation (TMS) has made it possible to probe the plasticity of the neural circuits involved in dystonias [79]. In that way, it has been established that all these focal dystonias are caused by a loss of inhibitory function at the spinal cord level, with the participation of several cortical networks [80]. Equally important, is the development of a recent model in rats to study the phenomenon, generally known as the dystonic rat (dt). The animal shows impairment in the protein caytaxin, associated with climbing fiber-Purkinje cell synapse impairments [81].

One striking feature of the disorder, however, is the lack of pathological evidence in human postmortem studies, thus implicating a dynamic circuit failure instead of an anatomical disability [82]. Consequently, dystonia can be associated with the development of defective plasticity in the striatum, with evidence indicating that acetylcholine and dopamine may be implicated (See [83] for a review). However, the search for a standard correlation between physiological findings and patients' clinical traits has been hampered due to differences in methodology and clinical characteristics of the enrolled population [84].

Nonetheless, it seems clear that, at least two factors concur to produce primary dystonia: a) repetitive use or injury of the affected body part and b) basal abnormal plastic mechanisms that predispose the development of dystonia [78, 85]. These factors, it is hypothesized, may converge to produce a deficient cortical plasticity driving the dystonic movements. It has been shown that overtraining monkeys in a repetitive motor task produces an abnormal rewiring of the somatosensory cortex [86]; with similar results in humans and rats [87].

Since direct recordings of human electrophysiological activity are rare, the use of transcranial magnetic stimulation (TMS), which offers a window on corticospinal excitability, has become an important technique. Based on these studies Quartarone et al [88] proposed a model on how dystonia may be produced in the corticostriatal synapses. In this system, high-frequency stimulation is able to produce Long Term Potentiation or Long Term Depression, depending on NMDA receptor activation. Under these conditions, a train of low-frequency stimulation could reverse LTP, a phenomenon known as depotentiation. However, these physiological changes occur accompanied by neuroanatomical changes, increasing or decreasing dendritic spines. In another model of dystonia, a knockout mice lacking torsinA in cortex and striatum, profound alterations of synaptic plasticity affect their motor behavior and motor learning. Due to the increased magnitude of LTP in these animals, depotentiation and LTD do not occur [89], pointing toward exacerbated plasticity that would lead to the development of symptoms observed in dystonia.

HOMEOSTATIC SYNAPTIC PLASTICITY

Homeostatic plasticity represents a negative feedback mechanism that evolved to limit the amount of excitation or inhibition experienced by a neural system and, in that way, maintain synaptic strength within specific (healthy) limits. Developing brains are more sensitive to homeostatic regulation, which is thought of as a protective mechanism against instability at a time when the system is under intense remodeling [90]. Interestingly, the mechanisms seem to depend on an intensification of NMDA receptors targeting, and associated with an increase in synaptic size [91]. Based on the evidence reviewed so far, these kind of concepts may be useful to understand and predict some of the observed effects on cortico-striatal plasticity failure.

One of the early models of homeostatic plasticity, proposed by McEachern and colleagues, pointed out that LTP and LTD could be seen as extremes in a continuum between plasticity and pathology [92]. The model proposed a relationship between LTP and kindling[1] on one side, and LTD on the other, while denying, however, that LTP is directly related to learning and memory. In this view, synaptic modifications rely on the age-dependent regulation of neurotransmitter receptors: homeostatic regulation would be a feature of adult systems in which the system compensates for changes in synaptic input; on the other hand, developing neural systems use a homeodynamic receptor regulation facilitating LTP and synaptogenesis in response to synaptic input. The nature of this synaptic input may be modulated by different elements such as "[...] intensity, frequency, duration, number of repetitions, level of postsynaptic depolarization, magnitude of rise in internal Ca2+, spatiotemporal pattern of stimulation, and [...] additional unknown factors" [92].

One of the main characteristics of the continuum model is that it identifies the margin on which plasticity is safely modulated, between LTP induction and LTD development, indicating that once high levels of excitation are reached beyond LTP, the system moves into a state of kindling that could lead to dangerous levels of excitotoxicity and even apoptotic degeneration (see figure 3A). It has been suggested that neurodegenerative processes may convert LTD into LTP and vice versa [32]. Parallel to this, other authors have suggested that the loss of synaptic homeostasis at cellular and system level could be the main factor leading to the motor dysfunction detected, for example, in dystonia [88].

One of the most influential models of homeostatic plasticity is the BCM theory. Originally proposed in 1982 by Bienenstock–Cooper–Munro [93], it was applied to neural development in the visual cortex. The rule was updated

---

[1] Kindling is a model of seizures characterized by what is called "afterdischarges" following high frequency stimulation. The afterdischarges subsequently have the tendency to spread on large areas of the brain.

more recently by Bear [94] and applied to glutamatergic synapses in hippocampus.

In short, the BCM rule proposes a "modification threshold" based on the interaction between presynaptic and postsynaptic activity: "presynaptic activity triggers synaptic depression or potentiation depending on the concurrent level of postsynaptic activity (i.e. the degree of correlation)" [94] (see figure 3B).

The Model Generally Pre dicts that:

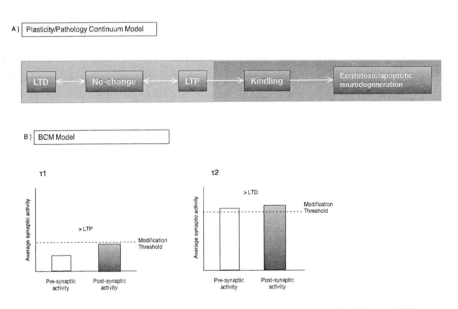

Figure 3. Two global models addressing the role of homeostatic plasticity. A) The Plasticity/Pathology Continuum proposed by McEachern (1996) expresses that LTD and LTP are two points in a scale that contains normal homeostatic plasticity (light green area). However, exceeding levels of excitability lead to epileptiform kindling and even excitotoxic neurodegeneration (dark grey area). B) The central element of the BCM theory is the presence of a modification threshold which varies according to the levels of averaged synaptic activity and we present, as an example, two possible scenarios: τ1) low levels of time-averaged postsynaptic activity increase the chances of LTP triggering; τ2) high levels of time-averaged postsynaptic activity increase the modification threshold, thus decreasing the probability for LTP induction. This, however, increases the chances of LTD induction. The use of average activity in the model demonstrates the importance of previous synaptic history in the current physiological state of the synapse.

1. LTD will occur in presynaptically active synapses when postsynaptic activity does not reach the modification threshold, although postsynaptical activity remains above zero;
2. When postsynaptic activity is low, the threshold is also low and the chances of triggering LTP increase - figure 3B, τ1;
3. An important consideration of the BCM model is that the threshold is not fixed, but is defined as time-variable. It changes depending on the history of the integrated postsynaptic activity. In this way, the threshold falls following low activity and it raises when activity levels increase - figure 3B, τ2.

A recent study by Muller and colleagues [95], supporting the BCM model through the application of paired associative stimulation (PAS), confirmed that a history of prior conditioning can modulate the LTP-like plasticity in human motor cortex (area M1). Using somatosensory motor evoked potentials (MEP) as an index of plasticity, the study compared two PAS sessions in eleven volunteers. During the first session, PAS was used to induce either an LTP-like increase, LTD-like decrease or no change. Subsequently, in a second session performed 30 minutes later, an LTP protocol was always applied. The MEPs, recorded from the right abductor pollicis brevis (APB) muscle, expressed a modest LTP only if no change has been induced in the previous session. However, the response increased if there was a previous history of LTD but it markedly dropped if the pathway has previously experimented LTP. This seems to be the only example of direct application of the models described above, particularly following homeostatic mechanisms as predicted by the BCM theory. Although these models may account for the physiological conditions that lead to plasticity failure, a more specific link with current data has not been established.

CONCLUSION

In previous sections we offered a concise survey pertaining to the relationship between plastic processes, like LTP and LTD, and their impairment in neurological diseases. We focused on human findings where considerable data indicates that an impairment of plastic processes is a common thread linking different neurological diseases such as Alzheimer's, Parkinson's, Huntington's and dystonia, both at the cellular and network level.

Although these diseases present different symptomatology and time-courses, the presence of synaptic anomalies is an striking feature that reclaims more in depth studies. However, the evidence so far does not point clearly to plastic mechanisms as a cause or a side effect, while few attempts exist to develop a theory with a unified mechanism of action. Recent advances seem to indicate that this common mechanism could be found through a deeper understanding of homeostatic plasticity. Since homeostasis is a central regulatory element in the CNS, it makes sense, from a neural perspective, to look at the variables that affect its normal functioning.

More recently, interest has increased in the area of homeostatic synaptic plasticity (see [96] for a recent review). Many cellular and molecular factors are currently being studied, including pre and postsynaptic mechanisms; activity-induced gene expression and local synthesis; secreted molecules such as neurotrophins as well as cytokines and cell adhesion molecules such as integrins. Homeostatic networks seem to depend on multiple mechanisms with striking variability in their temporal and spatial characteristics. In this sense, important differences have been pointed out between the heterogeneity of mechanisms observed in vivo versus the ones detected in dissociated cultures [96]. This is an area where the need for converging studies of the whole system, considering its intrinsic circuit modulation and specific outputs, together with cellular excitation and inhibition, will be played out in the future. It is likely that this multilevel approach could shed light on the association between homeostatic plasticity and pathology. However, few global approaches, like the ones represented by the plasticity-pathology continuum model and the BCM theory, actually exist.

Fortunately, some therapeutic approaches consider the enhancement of plasticity as an important element to improve cognitive performance. These approaches run the gamut from physiological to behavioral interventions, but all of them are intended to increase patients' quality of life. At a cellular level, we can cite some therapeutic approaches directed at enhancing axonal regeneration, reinnervation and general reorganization of the CNS [36], as well as proposing a deeper understanding of the role played by protective agents, such as nicotine [97]. At a more physiological level, deep brain stimulation (DBS) has proved effective in reducing motor symptoms in Parkinson's disease, dystonia and other maladies [98]. However, new non-invasive technologies like repetitive transcranial magnetic stimulation (rTMS) and transcranial direct current stimulation (tDCS) are becoming more popular, especially applied to the relief of symptoms from Parkinson's and dystonia, bringing beneficial effects by normalizing cortical excitability and increasing the release of dopamine [99]. Finally, at a behavioral level, enriched environments (EE) have been known to increase synaptic connectivity and enhance neurological function in animal models of Alzheimer's, Parkinson's and Huntington's disease [100]. Maybe the future will make clear that the synergy of these different technologies and approaches could produce the best results for the patients as well as increasing our understanding on the inner workings of the CNS.

REFERENCES

[1] Bliss T, Lømo T. Long-lasting potentiation of synaptic transmission in the dentate area of anaesthetized rabbit following stimulation of the perforant path. *Journal of Physiology.* 1973;232:331-56.
[2] Hebb DO. *The Organization of Behavior: A Neuropsychological Theory* New York: Lawrence Erlbaum; New edition; 1949.
[3] Lynch MA. Long-Term Potentiation and Memory. *Physiol Rev.* 2004 January 1, 2004;84(1):87-136.
[4] Cooke SF, Bliss TVP. Plasticity in the human central nervous system. *Brain.* 2006;129(7):1659-73.
[5] Abraham WC, Williams JM. Properties and mechanisms of LTP maintenance. *Neuroscientist.* 2003;9:463–74.
[6] Barrionuevo G, Schottler F, Lynch G. The effects of repetitive low frequency stimulation on control and "potentiated" synaptic responses in the hippocampus. *Life Sciences.* 1980;27(24):2385-91.
[7] McNaughton BL, Douglas RM, Goddard GV. Synaptic enhancement in fascia dentata: Cooperativity among coactive afferents. *Brain Research.* 1978;157(2):277-93.
[8] Barr D, Lambert N, Hoyt K, Moore S, Wilson W. Induction and Reversal of Long-Term Potentiation by Low- and High-Intensity Theta pattern Stimulation. *The Journal of Neuroscience.* 1995;15(7):5402-10.
[9] Collingridge GL, Bliss TVP. Memories of NMDA receptors and LTP. *Trends in Neurosciences.* 1995;18(2):54-6.
[10] Raymond CR. LTP forms 1, 2 and 3: different mechanisms for the 'long' in long-term potentiation. *Trends in Neurosciences.* 2007;30(4):167-75.
[11] Lynch G, Rex CS, Gall CM. LTP consolidation: Substrates, explanatory power, and functional significance. *Neuropharmacology.* 2007; 52(1):12-23.

[12] Whitlock JR, Heynen, A. J., Shuler, M.G., Bear, M.F. Learning induces Long-Term Potentiation in the Hippocampus. *Science.* 2006;313:1093-7.
[13] Teyler TJ, Cavus I, Coussens C. Synaptic plasticity in the hippocampal slice: functional consequences. *Journal of Neuroscience Methods.* 1995;59(1):11-7.
[14] Massey PV, Bashir ZI. Long-term depression: multiple forms and implications for brain function. *Trends in Neurosciences.* 2007;30(4):176-84.
[15] Jiao S, Li Z. Nonapoptotic Function of BAD and BAX in Long-Term Depression of Synaptic Transmission. *Neuron.* 2011;70(4):758-72.
[16] Rowan M. Stress and long-term synaptic depression. *Molecular Psychiatry.* 1998;3:472–4.
[17] Ahmed T, Sabanov V, D'Hooge R, Balschun D. An N-methyl-d-aspartate-receptor dependent, late-phase long-term depression in middle-aged mice identifies no GluN2-subunit bias. *Neuroscience.* 2011;185:27-38.
[18] Beck H, Goussakov IV, Lie A, Helmstaedter C, Elger CE. Synaptic plasticity in the human dentate gyrus. *Journal of Neuroscience.* 2000;20:7080-6.
[19] Chen WR, Lee S, Kato K, Spencer DD, Shepherd GM, Williamson A. Long-term modifications of synaptic efficacy in the human inferior and middle temporal cortex. *Proceedings of the National Academy of Science USA.* 1996;93:8011-5.
[20] Teyler TJ, Hamm J, Clapp WC, Jhonson B, Corballis M, Kirk IJ. Long-term Potentiation of Human Visual Evoked Responses. *European Journal of Neuroscience.* 2005;21:2045-50.
[21] Clapp WC, Kirk, I. J., Hamm, J. P., D. Shepherd and Teyler, T. J. Induction of LTP in the human auditory cortex by sensory stimulation. *European Journal of Neuroscience.* 2005;22:1135-40.
[22] Ross RM, McNair NA, Fairhall SL, Clapp WC, Hamm JP, Teyler TJ, et al. Induction of orientation-specific LTP-like changes in human visual evoked potentials by rapid sensory stimulation. *Brain Research Bulletin.* 2008;76(1-2):97-101.
[23] Battaglia F, Wang H-Y, Ghilardi MF, Gashi E, Quartarone A, Friedman E, et al. Cortical Plasticity in Alzheimer's Disease in Humans and Rodents. *Biological Psychiatry.* 2007;62(12):1405-12.

[24] Córdoba-Montoya DA, Albert J, López-Martín S. All together now: long term potentiation in the human cortex. *Rev Neurol.* 2010;51:367-74.
[25] Packard MG, Knowlton BJ. Learning and memory functions of the basal ganglia. *Annu Rev Neurosci.* 2002;25:563–93.
[26] Graybiel AM, Aosaki T, Flaherty AW, Kimura M. The basal ganglia and adaptive motor control. *Science.* 1994;265:1826–31.
[27] Jin X, Costa RM. Start/stop signals emerge in nigrostriatal circuits during sequence learning. *Nature.* 2010;466:457–62.
[28] Jog MS, Kubota Y, Connolly CI, Hillegaart V, Graybiel AM. Building neural representations of habits. *Science.* 1999;286:1745–9.
[29] Diamond DM, Fleshner M, Rose GM. Psychological stress repeatedly blocks hippocampal primed burst potentiation in behaving rats. *Behav Brain Res.* 1994;62:1-9.
[30] Diamond DM, Fleshner M, Ingersoll N, Rose GM. Psychological stress impairs spatial working memory: relevance to electrophysiological studies of hippocampal function. *Behav Neurosci* 1996;110:661– 72.
[31] Kim JJ, Diamond DM. The stressed hippocampus, synaptic plasticity and lost memories. *Nat Rev Neurosci.* 2002;3:453–62.
[32] Calabresi P, Galletti F, Saggese E, Ghiglieri V, Picconi B. Neuronal networks and synaptic plasticity in Parkinson's disease: beyond motor deficits. *Parkinsonism and Related Disorders.* 2007;13(Supplement 3):S259-S62.
[33] Kung VWS, Hassam R, Morton AJ, Jones S. Dopamine-dependent long term potentiation in the dorsal striatum is reduced in the R6/2 mouse model of Huntington's disease. *Neuroscience.* 2007;146(4):1571-80.
[34] Zuccato C, Cattaneo E. Role of brain-derived neurotrophic factor in Huntington's disease. *Progress in Neurobiology.* 2007;81(5-6):294-330.
[35] Crupi D, Ghilardi MF, Mosiello C, Di Rocco A, Quartarone A, Battaglia F. Cortical and brainstem LTP-like plasticity in Huntington's disease. *Brain Research Bulletin.* 2008;75(1):107-14.
[36] Navarro X, Vivo M, Valero-Cabre A. Neural plasticity after peripheral nerve injury and regeneration. *Progress in Neurobiology.* 2007;82(4):163-201.
[37] 2011 Alzheimer's disease facts and figures. *Alzheimer's and Dementia.* 2011;7(2):208-44.
[38] Hardy J, Selkoe DJ. The amyloid hypothesis of Alzheimer's disease: progress and problems on the road to therapeutics. *Science.* 2002;297:353-6.

[39] Findeis MA. The role of amyloid [beta] peptide 42 in Alzheimer's disease. *Pharmacology and Therapeutics.* 2007;116(2):266-86.

[40] Walsh DM, Klyubin I, Fadeeva JV, Cullen WK, Anwyl R, Wolfe MS, et al. Naturally secreted oligomers of amyloid beta protein potently inhibit hippocampal long-term potentiation in vivo. *Nature.* 2002;416:535-9.

[41] Wang HW, Pasternak JF, Kuo H, Ristic H, Lambert MP, Chromy B, et al. Soluble oligomers of [beta]amyloid (1-42) inhibit long- term potentiation but not long-term depression in rat dentate gyrus. *Brain Res.* 2002;924:133-40.

[42] Wang Q-w, Rowan MJ, Anwyl R. Inhibition of LTP by beta-amyloid is prevented by activation of [beta]2 adrenoceptors and stimulation of the cAMP/PKA signalling pathway. *Neurobiology of Aging.* 2009;30 (10):1608-13.

[43] Srivareerat M, Tran TT, Salim S, Aleisa AM, Alkadhi KA. Chronic nicotine restores normal A[beta] levels and prevents short-term memory and E-LTP impairment in A[beta]rat model of Alzheimer's disease. *Neurobiology of Aging.* 2011;32(5):834-44.

[44] Cook IA, Leuchter AF. Synaptic dysfunction in Alzheimer's disease: clinical assessment using quantitative EEG. *Behav Brain Res.* 1996;78:15-23.

[45] Koch G, Esposito Z, Codecà C, Mori F, Kusayanagi H, Monteleone F, et al. Altered dopamine modulation of LTD-like plasticity in Alzheimer's disease patients. *Clinical Neurophysiology.* 2011;122 (4):703-7.

[46] Yu J-T, Chang RC-C, Tan L. Calcium dysregulation in Alzheimer's disease: From mechanisms to therapeutic opportunities. *Progress in Neurobiology.* 2009;89(3):240-55.

[47] Cepeda C, Wu N, André VM, Cummings DM, Levine MS. The corticostriatal pathway in Huntington's disease. *Progress in Neurobiology.* 2007;81(5-6):253-71.

[48] Bates G, Harper P, Jones L. *Huntington's disease,* 3rd edition. Oxford: Oxford University Press; 2002.

[49] Johnson MA, Rajan V, Miller CE, Wightman RM. Dopamine release is severely compromised in the R6/2 mouse model of Huntington's disease. *J Neurochem.* 2006;97:737–46.

[50] Levine MS, Cepeda C, Hickey MA, Fleming SM, Chesselet MF. Genetic mouse models of Huntington's and Parkinson's diseases: illuminating but imperfect. *Trends in Neurosciences.* 2004;27:691–7.

[51] Smith R, Chung H, Rundquist S, Maat-Schieman ML, Colgan L, Englund E, et al. Cholinergic neuronal defect without cell loss in Huntington's disease. *Hum Mol Genet* 2006;15:3119–31.
[52] Ciamei A, Morton AJ. Rigidity in social and emotional memory in the R6/2 mouse model of Huntington's disease. *Neurobiology of Learning and Memory.* 2008;89(4):533-44.
[53] Berretta N, Nisticò R, Bernardi G, Mercuri NB. Synaptic plasticity in the basal ganglia: A similar code for physiological and pathological conditions. *Progress in Neurobiology.* 2008;84(4):343-62.
[54] Calabresi P, Pisani A, Mercuri NB, Bernardi G. The cortico-striatal projection: from synaptic plasticity to dysfunctions of the basal ganglia. *Trends Neurosci.* 1996;19:19–24.
[55] Fino E, Glowinski J, Venance L. Bidirectional activity-dependent plasticity at corticostriatal synapses. *J Neurosci.* 2005;25:11279–87.
[56] Fan MMY, Raymond LA. N-Methyl-d-aspartate (NMDA) receptor function and excitotoxicity in Huntington's disease. *Progress in Neurobiology.* 2007;81(5-6):272-93.
[57] Ferrante RJ, Kowall NW, Cipolloni PB, Storey E, Beal MF. Excitotoxin lesions in primates as a model for Huntington's disease: histopathologic and neurochemical characterization. *Exp Neurol* 1993;119:46-71.
[58] Coyle JT, Schwarcz R. Lesion of striatal neurons with kainic acid provides a model for Huntington's chorea. *Nature.* 1976;263:244–6.
[59] Gubellini P, Centonze D, Tropepi D, Bernardi G, Calabresi P. Induction of corticostriatal LTP by 3-nitropropionic acid requires the activation of mGluR1/PKC pathway. *Neuropharmacology.* 2004;46(6):761-9.
[60] Picconi B, Passino E, Sgobio C, Bonsi P, Barone I, Ghiglieri V, et al. Plastic and behavioral abnormalities in experimental Huntington's disease: A crucial role for cholinergic interneurons. *Neurobiology of Disease.* 2006;22(1):143-52.
[61] Stefan K, Kunesch E, Cohen LG, Benecke R, J. C. Induction of plasticity in the human motor cortex by paired associative stimulation. *Brain* 2000;123 (Pt 3) 572–84.
[62] Rajput AH. Environmental toxins accelerate Parkinson's disease onset. *Neurology.* 2001;56(1):4-5.
[63] Uitti RJ, Baba Y, Wszolek ZK, Putzke DJ. Defining the Parkinson's disease phenotype: initial symptoms and baseline characteristics in a clinical cohort. Parkinsonism andamp; *Related Disorders.* 2005;11(3):139-45.

[64] Miyake Y, Sasaki S, Tanaka K, Fukushima W, Kiyohara C, Tsuboi Y, et al. Dietary fat intake and risk of Parkinson's disease: A case-control study in Japan. *Journal of the Neurological Sciences.* 2010;288(1-2):117-22.

[65] Brassat D, Durr A, Agid Y, Brice A. Génétique de la maladie de Parkinson / Genetic aspect of Parkinson's disease. *La Revue de Médecine Interne.* 1999;20(8):709-14.

[66] Goberman AM, Blomgren M, Metzger E. Characteristics of speech disfluency in Parkinson disease. *Journal of Neurolinguistics.* 2010;23 (5):470-8.

[67] Kimmeskamp S, Hennig EM. Heel to toe motion characteristics in Parkinson patients during free walking. *Clinical Biomechanics.* 2001;16(9):806-12.

[68] Song I-U, Kim J-S, Jeong D-S, Song H-J, Lee K-S. Early neuropsychological detection and the characteristics of Parkinson's disease associated with mild dementia. *Parkinsonism andamp; Related Disorders.* 2008;14(7):558-62.

[69] Van Spaendonck KPM, Berger HJC, Horstink MWIM, Buytenhuijs EL, Cools AR. Executive functions and disease characteristics in Parkinson's disease. *Neuropsychologia.* 1996;34(7):617-26.

[70] Ungerstedt U. Postsynaptic supersensitivity after 6-hydroxydopamine induced degeneration of the nigro-striatal dopamine system. *Acta Physiol Scand.* 1971a;367:69–93.

[71] Ungerstedt U. Striatal dopamine release after amphetamine or nerve degeneration revealed by rotational behaviour. *Acta Physiol Scand.* 1971b;367:49–68.

[72] Schwarting RKW, Huston JP. The unilateral 6-hydroxydopamine lesion model in behavioral brain research, Analysis of func- tional deficits, recovery and treatments. *Prog Neurobiol.* 1996;50:275–331.

[73] Wiecki TV, Frank MJ. Neurocomputational models of motor and cognitive deficits in Parkinson's disease. In: Anders B, Cenci MA, editors. *Progress in Brain Research: Elsevier;* 2010. p. 275-97.

[74] Centonze D, Gubellini P, Picconi B, Calabresi P, Giacomini P, Bernardi G. Unilateral dopamine denervation blocks corticos- triatal LTP. *J Neurophysiol* 1999;82:3575–9.

[75] Ueki Y, Mima T, Ali Kotb M, Ikeda A, Sawada H, Fukuyama H, et al. Associative plasticity of the motor cortex in Parkinson's disease. *International Congress Series.* 2005;1278:299-302.

[76] Suppa A, Marsili L, Belvisi D, Conte A, Iezzi E, Modugno N, et al. Lack of LTP-like plasticity in primary motor cortex in Parkinson's disease. *Experimental Neurology.* 2011;227(2):296-301.
[77] Müller U. The monogenic primary dystonias. *Brain.* 2009;132:2005–25.
[78] Torres-Russotto D, Perlmutter JS. Task-specific dystonias: a review. *Ann NY Acad Sci.* 2008;1142:179–99.
[79] Rothwell J. Transcranial magnetic stimulation as a method for investigating the plasticity of the brain in Parkinson's Disease and dystonia. *Parkinsonism and Related Disorders.* 2007;13(Supplement 3):S417-S20.
[80] Hallett M. Neurophysiology of dystonia: The role of inhibition. *Neurobiology of Disease.* 2011;42(2):177-84.
[81] LeDoux MS. Animal models of dystonia: Lessons from a mutant rat. *Neurobiology of Disease.* 2011;42(2):152-61.
[82] Standaert DG. Update on the pathology of dystonia. *Neurobiol Dis.* 2011;42:148–51.
[83] Peterson DA, Sejnowski TJ, Poizner H. Convergent evidence for abnormal striatal synaptic plasticity in dystonia. *Neurobiology of Disease.* 2010;37(3):558-73.
[84] Tinazzi M, Squintani G, Berardelli A. Does neurophysiological testing provide the information we need to improve the clinical management of primary dystonia? *Clinical Neurophysiology.* 2009;120(8):1424-32.
[85] Altenmüller E, Jabusch HC. Focal dystonia in musicians: phenomenology, pathophysiology and triggering factors. *Eur J Neurol.* 2010;17(Suppl. 1):31–6.
[86] Byl NN, Merzenich MM, Jenkins WM. A primate genesis model of focal dystonia and repetitive strain injury: I. Learning-induced dedifferentiation of the representation of the hand in the primary somatosensory cortex in adult monkeys. *Neurology.* 1996;47:508–20.
[87] Godde B, Spengler F, Dinse HR. Associative pairing of tactile stimulation induces somatosensory cortical reorganization in rats and humans. *NeuroReport.* 1996;8(1):281-5.
[88] Quartarone A, Pisani A. Abnormal plasticity in dystonia: Disruption of synaptic homeostasis. *Neurobiology of Disease.* 2011;42(2):162-70.
[89] Martella G, Tassone A, Sciamanna G, Platania P, Cuomo D, Viscomi MT, et al. Impairment of bidirectional synaptic plasticity in the striatum of a mouse model of DYT1 dystonia: role of endogenous acetylcholine. *Brain.* 2009;132:2336–49.

[90] Huupponen J, Molchanova SM, Taira T, Lauri SE. Susceptibility for homeostatic plasticity is down-regulated in parallel with maturation of the rat hippocampal synaptic circuitry. *The Journal of Physiology.* 2007 Jun 1;581(Pt 2):505-14.
[91] Carpenter-Hyland EP, Chandler LJ. Adaptive plasticity of NMDA receptors and dendritic spines: Implications for enhanced vulnerability of the adolescent brain to alcohol addiction. *Pharmacology Biochemistry and Behavior.* 2007;86(2):200-8.
[92] McEachern JC, Shaw CA. An alternative to the LTP orthodoxy: a plasticity-pathology continuum model. *Brain Research Reviews.* 1996;22(1):51-92.
[93] Bienenstock EL, Cooper LN, Munro PW. Theory for the development of neuron selectivity: orientation specificity and binocular interaction in visual cortex. *J Neurosci.* 1982;2:32–48.
[94] Bear MF. Bidirectional synaptic plasticity: from theory to reality. *Philos Trans R Soc Lond B Biol Sci.* 2003;358:649–55.
[95] Müller JFM, Orekhov Y, Liu Y, Ziemann U. Homeostatic plasticity in human motor cortex demonstrated by two consecutive sessions of paired associative stimulation. *European Journal of Neuroscience.* 2007;25(11):3461-8.
[96] Pozo K, Goda Y. Unraveling mechanisms of homeostatic synaptic plasticity. *Neuron.* 2010 May 13;66(3):337-51.
[97] Welsby PJ, Rowan MJ, Anwyl R. Beta-amyloid blocks high frequency stimulation induced LTP but not nicotine enhanced LTP. *Neuropharmacology.* 2007;53(1):188-95.
[98] Gubellini P, Salin P, Kerkerian-Le Goff L, Baunez C. Deep brain stimulation in neurological diseases and experimental models: From molecule to complex behavior. *Progress in Neurobiology.* 2009;89(1):79-123.
[99] Wu AD, Fregni F, Simon DK, Deblieck C, Pascual-Leone A. Noninvasive Brain Stimulation for Parkinson's Disease and Dystonia. *Neurotherapeutics.* 2008;5(2):345-61.
[100] Wood NI, Glynn D, Morton AJ. "Brain training" improves cognitive performance and survival in a transgenic mouse model of Huntington's disease. *Neurobiology of Disease.* 2011;42(3):427-37.

In: Synaptic Plasticity
Editors: G. N. McMahon et al.

ISBN: 978-1-62081-004-0
© 2012 Nova Science Publishers, Inc.

Chapter V

SYNAPTIC PLASTICITY IN ADDICTION[*]

Yan Dong[1,†] *and R. Suzanne Zukin*[2]

[1]Department of Vet and Comparative Anatomy, Pharmacology and Physiology, Washington State University, Pullman, US
[2]Department of Neuroscience, Albert Einstein College of Medicine, Bronx, NY, US

ABSTRACT

Drug addiction, defined as compulsive drug use despite serious negative consequences, has been one of the major social problems facing modern societies. A growing body of evidence suggests that drug exposure induces a series of adaptive changes within the brain reward circuitry, some of which are extremely long-lasting and which may mediate maladaptive emotion/reward learning and memory, thus leading to addiction. Here, we review recent findings concerning drug-induced neuronal plasticity occurring at excitatory synapses in the brain areas that make up the reward circuitry. Given that the synapse plays a critical role in neuronal plasticity, drug-induced synaptic plasticity may critically mediate the formation of drug-related memories and thereby, addictive behaviors.

---

[*] A version of this chapter also appears in *Cognitive Science Compendium. Volume 1*, edited by Miao-Kun Sun, published by Nova Science Publishers, Inc. It was submitted for appropriate modifications in an effort to encourage wider dissemination of research.
[†] Correspondence. E-mail: yandong@vetmed.wsu.edu.

1. INTRODUCTION

Acute exposure to addictive drugs usually produces an intensely positive affective state, or "high", which may lead to chronic drug use. After repeated drug exposure, a subpopulation of people develop addiction, manifested as compulsive drug use despite serious negative consequences including, for example, illness, disrupted personal relationships and failures in major life roles (Hyman and Malenka, 2001). Over the past two decades considerable efforts have been devoted to elucidating the neuronal mechanisms of drug addiction. Given that addictive drugs are usually rewarding and motivating, early attention was intuitively focused on brain circuits of the co-called the "reward pathway" which, under normal conditions, mediates natural rewards (such as food, drink and sex) and reward-associated emotion/motivation (Wise and Bozarth, 1987). As originally defined, the reward pathway includes the midbrain ventral tegmental area (VTA) and the nucleus accumbens (NAc), which receives dopaminergic innervation from the VTA, and which provides reciprocal inhibitory (GABAergic) afferents to and from the VTA. Subsequent work has expanded the reward pathways by including a number of several related neuroanatomic regions, such as the prefrontal cortex, the hippocampal formation and the amygdala.

The brain reward pathway mediates reward/emotion/motivation learning and memory. Unlike the classroom learning and memory that we are consciously aware of, reward/emotion/motivation learning and memory can happen subconsciously, which is perceived but implicit. For example for individuals who previously have experienced frightening car accidents, a glance at a related cue (same brand of car or similar street corner) can instantly elicit an entire panoply of emotions including strong fear and increased heart rate, before the explicit memory is recalled. The fearful emotional state is learned and stored as a memory that can be wakened by associated cues to produce behavioral consequences such as running away from the emotion-eliciting site. The normophysiologic process mediated by the reward pathway can be usurped by addictive drugs to produce a state of addiction. Exposure to addictive drugs induces an extremely strong and long-lasting pathological emotional memory that, once awakened, manifests as a robust sense of craving.

An abundance of evidence suggests that the process by which addictive drugs produce persistent alterations in brain function may share common molecular and cellular mechanisms with experience-dependent neuronal plasticity at excitatory synapses of key brain regions such as the VTA and

NAc (Kelley, 2004; Wolf et al., 2004). As such, one of the major goals of the field is to identify drug-induced neuronal plasticity in the brain reward pathway, with the hope that such efforts may result in the identification of critical maladaptive neuronal plasticity that leads to addiction. Given the leading role of the excitatory synapse in neuronal plasticity, in this review we focus on drug-induced plasticity occurring at excitatory synapses in the brain reward pathway.

2. SYNAPTIC PLASTICITY

Synaptic plasticity, or more precisely, experience-dependent changes in the efficacy or strength of synaptic transmission, plays a critical role in formation of memories (Bear, 1996). The most intensely studied and well-known cellular models of synaptic plasticity are long-term potentiation (LTP), or the persistent increase in the strength of synaptic transmission, and long-term depression (LTD), or the persistent decrease in the strength of synaptic transmission (Malenka and Nicoll, 1999). There are several different forms of LTP and LTD with very different molecular mechanisms, among which the best characterized are LTP and LTD at hippocampal CA1 synapses.

Two relevant glutamate receptor types, the alpha-amino-3-hydroxy-5-methyl-4-isoxazole propionic acid (AMPA) receptor and the N-methyl-D-aspartate (NMDA) receptor, are expressed at most excitatory synapses of hippocampal CA1 neurons. Binding of presynaptically-released glutamate is sufficient for the activation of AMPA receptors and conduction of a depolarizing current, rendering the postsynaptic neuron more likely to fire action potentials. However, NMDA receptor activation requires not only the binding of glutamate but also strong depolarization of the postsynaptic membrane to relieve the magnesium blockade of the channel pore. Unlike AMPA receptors, which mainly flux sodium (Na+) ions, activated NMDA receptors readily conduct calcium (Ca2+) ions into the postsynaptic cell. It is this NMDA receptor-dependent calcium influx that acts, via multiple intracellular signaling pathways, to trigger both LTP and LTD, respectively (Malenka and Nicoll, 1999). More specifically, depending on the intracellular level and spatial compartmentalization, calcium ions can either activate either protein kinases (e.g. calcium/calmodulin-dependent protein kinase II, or CaMKII) or protein phosphotases (e.g. calcium/calmodulin-dependent protein phosphatase calcineurin and protein phosphatase 1, or PP1) (Malinow and Malenka, 2002). CaMKII appears to trigger the delivery of intracellular

AMPA receptors to the postsynaptic membrane surface, producing LTP, whereas PPI and/or calcineurin can induce internalization of the AMPA receptors from the postsynaptic membrane, and thus produce LTD (Malenka, 2003). Thus the strength of the excitatory synapses will be persistently upregulated (LTP) when the number of postsynaptic AMPA receptors is increased and persistently downregulated (LTD) when the number of postsynaptic AMPA receptors is decreased.

AMPA receptors are tetramers composed of combinations of subunits including GluR1, GluR2, GluR3 and in the early developmental stage also Glu4 (Malinow and Malenka, 2002). Each subunit contains a unique intracellular C-terminal that selectively interacts with different binding partners and may activate different intracellular signaling cascades and, as such, is subject to differential regulation during LTP and LTD. For example, GluR1 appears to be essential for LTP, as hippocampal LTP is absent either in GluR1 knock out animals (Zamanillo et al., 1999) and or when the interaction between the GluR1 C-terminus and intracellular signaling cascades is interrupted (Shi et al., 1999). The molecular mechanisms of hippocampal LTD and LTD have been used as a template for synaptic plasticity study in other brain regions.

3. SYNAPTIC PLASTICITY IN THE BRAIN REWARD PATHWAY

As the backbone of the brain reward pathway, the mesocorticolimic dopamine (DA) system comprises the VTA, the NAc and the PFC (Tzschentke, 2001). This pathway mediates natural reinforcement as well as in the reinforcing properties of addictive drugs (Wise and Bozarth, 1987; Tzschentke, 2001). The VTA contains DA-releasing neurons, which project to the NAc and the PFC, and which receive excitatory projections from the PFC, the pedunculopontine nucleus and the bed nucleus of the stria terminalis (Tzschentke, 2001). The PFC sends glutamatergic projections to the VTA and the NAc. The major cell type of the NAc is the inhibitory GABAergic medium spiny neurons, which receive excitatory projections from the PFC, the hippocampus and the amygdala (Tzschentke, 2001). NAc cells are for the most part quiescent and their activity depends on excitatory input from cortical and subcortical limbic afferents (Nicola et al., 2000).

It is well documented that synaptic plasticity in the brain reward pathway share many core features in common with, but also distinctly different from that of hippocampal CA1 neurons. Excitatory synapses on neurons in the brain reward pathway can undergo both LTP and LTD. As in the hippocampus, LTP at excitatory synapses on VTA DA neurons requires activation of NMDA receptors (Bonci and Malenka, 1999), although it remains unclear as to whether CaMKII is the downstream effector (or target) of NMDA receptor-mediated calcium influx. LTD at excitatory synapses on VTA DA neurons, however, does not require activation of NMDA receptors but rather appears to be triggered by voltage-dependent calcium channels (Jones and Kauer, 1999; Thomas et al., 2000; Gutlerner et al., 2002). In addition, expression of LTD within VTA DA neurons involves regulated internalization of postsynaptic AMPA receptors, a process involving cAMP and activation of protein kinase A (PKA), but not activation of protein phosphatases 1/2A (Gutlerner et al., 2002).

Similar in VTA DA neurons, LTP can be induced in NAc neurons in an NMDA receptor-dependent manner and is likely expressed by upregulation of the postsynaptic AMPA receptor function/number (Kombian and Malenka, 1994). LTD in NAc neurons appears to be more complicated. Thus far there are two forms of LTD have been observed in NAc neurons: (1) NMDA receptor-dependent LTD, involving NMDA receptor mediated calcium influx and removal of postsynaptic AMPA receptors (Thomas et al., 2000); and (2) CB1 receptor-dependent LTD, in which endocannabinoind-mediated negative feedback causes a long-lasting depression of presynaptic glutamate release (Robbe et al., 2002b).

Current evidence suggests that both LTD and LTP can also be induced in the PFC neurons. LTP in PFC neurons requires activation of the NMDA receptor, whereas LTD appears to be NMDA receptor-independent and probably involves the CB1 receptor and metabotropic glutamate receptors (Huang et al., 2004). Since both the NAc and PFC receive dense DA projections, it is not surprising that DA plays a critical role in modulating the development and/or maintenance of synaptic plasticity in these two brain regions (Law-Tho et al., 1995; Otani et al., 1998; Gurden et al., 2000; Otani, 2003; Huang et al., 2004).

4. DRUG-INDUCED SYNAPTIC PLASTICITY IN THE BRAIN REWARD PATHWAY

Ventral Tegmental Area

There are two major cell types in the VTA, dopaminergic neurons and inhibitory GABA neurons, both of which project to target areas such as the NAc and PFC (Tzschentke, 2001). The neuronal activity of DA neurons is thought to encode information about the rewarding and motivationallly relevant properties of external stimuli and thus particularly important for the development of drug-induced addictive behaviors (Overton and Clark, 1997; Schultz, 2002). Glutamatergic afferents from the PFC and other limbic areas synapse on DA and GABA neurons in the VTA and importantly modulate the neuronal activity of VTA DA cells (Overton and Clark, 1997).

A critical question has been whether drugs of abuse induce long lasting synaptic plasticity in the brain reward pathway. Since LTP and LTD may involve insertion/internalization of AMPA receptors to/from the postsynaptic membrane, several early studies focused on the effects of drug of abuse on GluR1 protein levels within the VTA. A number of studies reported that repeated administration of cocaine, morphine (Fitzgerald et al., 1996) or ethanol (Ortiz et al., 1995) results in an increase in the level of the GluR1 subunit of AMPA glutamate receptors in the VTA. Other groups, however, found that there was no net change in GluR1 levels following cocaine or amphetamine administration (Lu et al., 2002). Since these studies used different schedules of drug administration, inconsistencies in their findings may reflect the fact that drug effects critically depend on the type of drug and the regimen of drug administration. It is worth noting that in most neurons there is a significant intracellular pool of AMPA receptors, and that expression studies of GluR1 transcript or protein levels alone may fail to reveal functionally important alterations in receptor trafficking. To directly assess the effects of drugs of abuse on VTA AMPA receptors, White and colleagues performed extracellular electrophysiological recording in living animals and observed that repeated cocaine or amphetamine exposure caused VTA DA neurons to be more responsive to iontophoresed AMPA (White et al., 1995). This important result can be interpreted as physiological evidence of an "LTP" like phenomena in VTA DA neurons following drug exposure. However, the direct physiological measurement in the above study is the AMPA receptor-evoked action potential bursting, not the synaptic AMPA receptor-mediate

EPSCs *per se*. It remains unclear whether the increased responsiveness occurs as a consequence of regulated AMPA receptor trafficking, and/or as a result of modulation of voltage-dependent ion channels, which are also important in synaptic responses to excitatory stimulation.

To directly assess the effects of drugs of abuse on the excitatory synaptic strength at VTA DA neurons, a series of studies have been conducted to measure the ratio of AMPA receptor-mediated synaptic current to NMDA receptor mediated synaptic current. This approach is predicted on the premise that LTP and LTD occur as a result of modification of synaptic AMPA receptor function/number, while the NMDA receptor function/number during LTP and LTD is relatively stable. Thus LTP is accompanied by an increase in the AMPA/NMDA ratio, whereas LTD is accompanied by a decrease in the AMPA/NMDA ratio. Therefore if a stimulus (e.g. administration of a drug of abuse) increases or decreases the AMPA/NMDA ratio, it is likely that this treatment may induce an LTP- or LTD-like process, accordingly. This approach offers the important advantage that it is independent of the number of synapses activated and therefore independent of such variables as the positioning of the electrodes or anatomy of the tissue.

Using this approach, Ungless et al., observed a substantial increase the AMPA/NMDA ratio in VTA DA neurons in acute brain slices prepared from animals receiving a single cocaine administration (Ungless et al., 2001). This cocaine-induced increase in the AMPA/NMDA ratio was abolished either in GluR1 (-/-) knockout mice or when NMDA receptors were selectively blocked by co-administration of the NMDA receptor antagonist MK801 (Ungless et al., 2001; Dong et al., 2004). Moreover, the ability to further enhance AMPA receptor mediated EPSCs (LTP induction) was diminished, whereas the ability to decrease the AMPA receptor-mediated EPSCs (LTD induction) was increased in VTA DA neurons from animals previously treated with cocaine, consistent with the idea that cocaine exposure, through an LTP-like process has already potentiated the AMPA receptor-mediated EPSCs. Taken together, these results indicate that *in vivo* cocaine administration induces a form of plasticity at excitatory synapses on midbrain DA neurons having in common many of the core features of hippocampal LTP.

Time course studies provide important clues regarding the behavioral correlates of this drug-induced synaptic adaptation. Cocaine-induced "LTP" in VTA DA neurons appears to have a fast onset and is relatively transient. It can be detected as soon as two hours after *in vivo* drug administration (Faleiro et al., 2004), and persists for at least five, but no more than ten, days (Ungless et al., 2001). The duration of the potentiation is also independent of the paradigm of cocaine treatment as the AMPA/NMDA ratio returns to the basal levels within ten days following the cessation of prolonged cocaine treatment (Borgland et al., 2004). Both the early onset and the relatively brief duration of drug-induced VTA "LTP" are consistent with the notion that this plasticity functions to prime the initial addictive processes, but are not the neuronal substrate for the long-term maintenance of the addicted state (Kalivas, 2004).

To further address whether the synaptic modification of VTA DA neurons is a mechanism specific to cocaine or, rather, is more generally applicable to all drugs of abuse, two subsequent studies (Saal et al., 2003; Dong et al., 2004) examined the effects of five addictive drugs: cocaine, amphetamine, morphine, nicotine and ethanol as well as two non-addictive psychoactive drugs Prozac (fluoxetine) and carbamazepine. The addictive drugs differ markedly in their *in vivo* triggering mechanisms. Cocaine and amphetamine acutely enhance DA transmission by blocking or reversing DA transporters. Morphine acutely activates opioid receptors; nicotine acutely activates nicotinic receptors. Ethanol acutely enhances GABAergic transmission. But they have one thing in common: they all cause addiction. The two control drugs are psychoactive and share some pharmacological effects with addictive drugs but do not cause addiction. For example, like cocaine and amphetamine, fluoxetine is a monoamine reuptake inhibitor, whereas carbamazepine like cocaine, blocks sodium channels. When administered *in vivo*, all five addictive drugs, but not the non-addictive drugs, increased the AMPA/NMDA ratio in VTA DA neurons (Saal et al., 2003). These findings suggest that this form of experience-dependent synaptic modification is specific for addictive drugs.

Stress is critically involved in addictive behaviors (Marinelli and Piazza, 2002; Shaham et al., 2003). Stress potentiates the acquisition of self-administration (Kabbaj et al., 2001), triggers reinstatement (Piazza and Le Moal, 1998), enhances conditioned place preference (CPP), and induces reinstatement of drug-seeking behaviors following extinction (Will et al., 1998; Sanchez and Sorg, 2001; Sanchez et al., 2003). Moreover, single exposure to stress increases the AMPA/NMDA ratio in VTA DA neurons in a manner similar to drugs of abuse (Saal et al., 2003). The stress- and cocaine-elicited effects on synaptic scaling exhibit mutual occlusion, and are both blocked by the NMDA receptor antagonist MK801. On the other hand, cocaine-, but not stress- induced synaptic potentiation in VTA DA neurons is blocked by DA D1-like antagonists, whereas the converse is true for glucocorticoid receptor blockade (Dong et al., 2004). Together, these findings indicate that whereas the *in vivo* triggering mechanisms for these forms of experience-dependent plasticity share some features in common, they differ in several important aspects (Dong et al., 2004).

The direct consequence of short-term LTP in VTA DA neurons following withdrawal from drug exposure is the enhancement of DA transmission. Enhanced DA transmission can be interpreted as an increase in the incentive salience attributed to drugs and drug-related cues, which may be experimentally manifested as behavioral sensitization (Robinson and Berridge, 2000). In parallel, VTA DA neurons may also function to establish and maintain the prediction of the reinforcing effect (e.g. reward) from the conditioned cues (Schultz, 2002) and are thus critically involved in conditioned behaviors related to addiction and reward.

Behavioral sensitization to drugs is an animal model for the intensification of drug craving, a core component of addiction. Behavioral sensitization arises during repeated drug administration and persists even after long periods of withdrawal (Robinson and Becker, 1986). This addiction-related behavior is highly conditional, as animals exhibiting higher levels of sensitization when exposed to the same environmental context in which their previous drug experience occurred (Badiani and Robinson, 2004). Another model for studying conditioned drug behavior is called conditioned place preference (CPP), in which animals show a strong preference for the place associated with drug experience.

Glutamatergic afferents on DA cells in the VTA are thought to be critical to several aspects of addictive behaviors, including behavioral sensitization and relapse to cocaine self-administration. In accordance with the general cognitive function of DA, it has been proposed that glutamatergic afferents to the NAc and cocaine-induced "LTP" in VTA DA neurons may play a critical role in cocaine induced behavioral sensitization, cocaine-conditioned sensitization, cocaine-induced CPP and relapse to cocaine self-administration. Indeed, this prevailing notion (Overton et al., 1999; Vanderschuren and Kalivas, 2000; Wolf et al., 2004) has been supported by many results. For example, intra VTA injection of NMDA receptor antagonist, which blocks drug-induced "LTP", blocks the induction of behavioral sensitization (Wolf, 1998) as well as CPP in response to cocaine administration (Kim et al., 1996; Harris and Aston-Jones, 2003). Animals with higher cocaine-induced AMPA/NMDA ratio in the VTA DA neurons exhibit a higher level of locomotor sensitization (Borgland et al., 2004). After discontinuing repeated psychostimulant administration, the VTA DA neurons remain superactive for several days, a time course consistent with that of cocaine-induced increases in the AMPA/NMDA ratio (White et al., 1995). This relatively transient superactivity of VTA DA neurons has been regarded as part of the mechanism that mediates "transfer" from the induction to the expression phase of locomotor sensitization (Wolf et al., 2004). In the case of CPP, it has been demonstrated that overexpression of GluR1 in the VTA causes a significant enhancement in morphine-induced CPP, while overexpression of GluR2, an AMPA receptor subunit not required for LTP, does not (Carlezon et al., 2001; Carlezon and Nestler, 2002). The role of VTA "LTP" in CPP is further suggested by the finding that the same dose of DA D1 receptor antagonist that blocks cocaine induced "LTP" in the VTA (Dong et al., 2004) blocks cocaine-induced CPP (Nazarian et al., 2004).

To directly examine whether the VTA "LTP" is required for cocaine-induced sensitization and CPP, we conducted a series of behavioral experiments using GluR1(-/-) knockout mice (Dong et al., 2004). These mice do not exhibit cocaine-induced potentiation of excitatory synaptic transmission (cocaine-induced "LTP") in VTA DA neurons. Surprisingly, the GluR1(-/-) knockout mice exhibit a robust behavioral sensitization to cocaine (Dong et al., 2004). This finding indicates that cocaine-induced LTP is not required for this form of behavioral plasticity. On the other hand, it remains unknown whether LTP in the VTA may contribute to the attribution of incentive value (motivational significance) to drug-related cues. While GluR1 deletion did not abolish sensitization to cocaine, two other behaviors were impaired in the knockout mice (Dong et al., 2004). The knockout mice did not exhibit cocaine-induced CPP. Moreover, the GluR1 knockout mice did not exhibit context-dependent enhancement of locomotor activity when placed in a conditioning apparatus in which they had received cocaine 24 hours previously (Dong et al., 2004). Cocaine-elicited LTP in VTA DA cells and CPP (Nazarian et al., 2004), as well as context-dependent enhancement of locomotor activity (Dong et al., 2004) were blocked by the same dose of a D1 receptor antagonist. Furthermore, both the cocaine-induced LTP in VTA DA cells and the cocaine-primed enhancement of morphine CPP (Kim et al., 2004) last five, but not ten, days (Borgland et al., 2004), and both can be blocked by an NMDA receptor antagonist. Taken collectively, these studies indicate that cocaine-induced LTP in VTA DA neurons may contribute to context-dependent associative learning and may contribute to attribution of incentive value (motivational significance) to drug-associated cues. More generally, since enhanced strength of excitatory synaptic strength in midbrain DA neurons will cause increased activities in DA cells (Overton and Clark, 1997; Grillner and Mercuri, 2002) and a consequent increase in DA release in target regions such as the NAc, experiences such as acute stress, which elicit LTP in the VTA may prime the animal such that subsequent experiences have greater incentive or motivational value.

Nucleus Accumbens

The NAc together with the VTA are the major components of the reward circuitry. Long-term changes in synaptic strength at excitatory synapses on NAc medium spiny neurons are critically important for many addictive behaviors. Early in situ hybridization and immunolabeling studies demonstrate that levels of GluR1 and GluR2 mRNA and protein are decreased in animals 14 days following withdrawal of repeated amphetamine administration (Lu et al., 1997; Lu et al., 1999; Lu and Wolf, 1999), whereas upregulation of GluR1 (but not GluR2) protein was also observed in the NAc of animals 30 days after withdrawal from repeated cocaine administration (Churchill et al., 1999). In the late 1990s White and his colleagues used extracellular recording combined with microiontophoretic techniques to measure glutamate-elicited action potential firing in NAc neurons and demonstrated that NAc neurons became hyposensitive to glutamate after withdrawal from chronic exposure to either cocaine or amphetamine (White et al., 1995). These results, while suggestive that drug exposure may elicit a postsynaptically- expressed LTD in the NAc, nevertheless have several possible caveats. For example, downregulation of mRNA levels of GluR1/2 does not necessarily correlate with downregulation of GluR1/2 protein, and may not be indicative of a downregulation of synaptic AMPA receptors. Furthermore, the reduced electrophysiological responses of NAc neurons are assessed by measuring action potential firing, which in addition to being mediated by metabotropic glutamate receptors, is also influenced by the activities of voltage-gated sodium, potassium and calcium channels, all of which may operate independently of glutamate receptor activities. Indeed, it has been demonstrated that exposure to cocaine persistently reduces both sodium (Zhang et al., 1998) and calcium currents (Zhang et al., 2002) in NAc neurons, changes that can attenuate neuronal excitability.

More recently, Thomas et al., showed that repetitive cocaine administration produces a decrease in the AMPA/NMDA ratio in NAc neurons (Thomas et al., 2001), consistent with a reduction in AMPA receptor number/function in the postsynaptic membrane and LTD. Furthermore, cocaine pretreatment enhances the amplitude of AMPA receptor miniature EPSCs, reduces the ability to generate LTD (Thomas et al., 2001) and increases the ability to generate LTP (Yao et al., 2004) in NAc neurons, implying that synaptic strength has been previously depressed by chronic drug exposure. Interestingly, exposure to amphetamine, another psychostimulant that shares similar molecular mechanismss of action with cocaine, does not alter NAc LTP (Li and Kauer, 2004).

Although the exact molecular mechanisms underlying drug-induced LTD in NAc neurons are as yet unknown, the available evidence suggests that DA may be critically involved in the induction phase of LTD. Unlike neurons of the dorsal striatum, DA is not required in the induction in vitro of LTD and LTP in NAc neurons (Pennartz et al., 1993; Thomas et al., 2000). Rather, DA, the selective DA D1 receptor agonist SKF82958 and the indirect agonist amphetamine all block tetanus-induced LTP (Li and Kauer, 2004). Moreover, cocaine exposure elevates the sensitivity of the D1 receptor in the NAc to endogenous and exogenous agonists (Beurrier and Malenka, 2002). It is tempting to speculate that excitatory synaptic strength in NAc neurons is constitutively modulated by endogenous factors such as DA and is finely balanced between potentiation and depression. Chronic drug administration enhances DA tone and thereby suppresses potentiation, thus shifting the equilibrium towards depression. This model predicts that any elevation of DA tone, even in the absence of drug administration, should also produce "LTD" in NAc neurons. Indeed, a recent finding indicates that excitatory synapses appear to be pre-depressed in the NAc slices from animals lacking DA transporters, norepinephrine transporters, or vesicular monoamine transporters, and that LTP of a greater magnitude could be induced (Yao et al., 2004). Clearly, more experiments are required to elucidate the role of DA in drug-induced NAc "LTD". An important unanswered question is whether direct microinjection of selective DA D1 receptor agonists can mimic, or whether antagonists can block, cocaine-induced "LTD" in NAc neurons.

Although the detailed molecular processes underlying the expression of drug-induced NAc LTD are also unclear, regulated glutamate receptor trafficking represents an intriguing model supported by a growing body of evidence. Recent studies show that repeated cocaine exposure reduces the levels of PSD-95 (Yao et al., 2004), a postsynaptic scaffolding protein that may control the AMPA receptor trafficking. Overexpression of PSD-95 increases the number of synaptic AMPA receptor and basal AMPA receptor mediated EPSC, occludes LTP and enhances LTD (Schnell et al., 2002; Beique and Andrade, 2003; Stein et al., 2003), whereas reduction of PSD-95 level decreases the number of synaptic AMPA receptors and the AMPA receptor mediated EPSCs (Nakagawa et al., 2004). Consistent with these findings, targeted disruption of PSD-95 abolishes LTD and facilitates the induction of LTP (Migaud et al., 1998; Komiyama et al., 2002). It has also been shown that controlling the availability and stability of PSD-95 by either ubiquitination or palmitoylation may serve as a mechanism to regulate the expression and maintenance of surface AMPA receptors (El-Husseini Ael et al., 2002; Colledge et al., 2003). It is conceivable that PSD-95 may play a similar role in the NAc, and thus diminished PSD-95 levels could contribute to cocaine-induced decreases in synaptic strength. It would be interesting to know whether cocaine exposure also affects the level of SAP97, the ubiquitination and/or palmitoylation of PSD-95, and whether cocaine-induced NAc "LTD" exists in PSD-95 null animals.

While the above observations indicate that drug exposure generates postynaptically-expressed LTD in NAc neurons, they do not exclude several other possible means by which drugs of abuse could alter synaptic strength. Evidence suggests that drug exposure may also modulate excitatory synaptic strength via presynaptic mechanisms. For example, DA presynaptically modulates excitatory synaptic transmission (Nicola et al., 2000). This presynaptic modulation is significantly enhanced by cocaine exposure (Beurrier and Malenka, 2002), and repeated cocaine administration decreases glutamate immunolabeling within the nerve terminals of the NAc shell (Keys et al., 1998; Meshul et al., 1998), suggesting enhanced presynaptic neurotransmitter release. In addition to evidence that addictive drugs can enhance presynaptic release, presynaptically expressed LTD, observed in both the NAc and dorsal striatum (Gerdeman et al., 2002; Robbe et al., 2002a), is blocked by the administration of a single dose of THC (Mato et al., 2004) or cocaine (Fourgeaud et al., 2004), suggesting that drugs of abuse can also modify the synaptic strength via presynaptic mechanisms.

Long-term changes in excitatory synaptic transmission, such as drug-induced "LTD", have been proposed to be critically involved in addiction-related behaviors (Wolf et al., 2004). This notion is supported by several behavioral studies. For example, intra-NAc infusion of NMDA receptor antagonists, which block several forms of synaptic plasticity, prevent the expression of behavioral sensitization (Li et al., 1997), the establishment of reinforcement learning (Kelley et al., 1997) and the acquisition (but not performance) of cue-elicited reinstatement of drug intake (McFarland and Kalivas, 2001; Park et al., 2002). Unfortunately so far there is no study directly describing the behavioral significance of cocaine-induced "LTD" in the NAc, but emerging evidence has started to provide clues that this form of plasticity may critically contribute to cocaine reward and behavioral sensitization. As shown by Kelz et al., (Kelz et al., 1999), overexpression of GluR1 in the NAc, the opposite to cocaine-induced "LTD", produces cocaine aversion. By analogy, NAc LTD may contribute to the enhancement of the incentive value of cocaine following repeated exposure. Consistent with this concept, blockade of calcineurin activity by the selective inhibitor FK506, a treatment that may interfere with the LTD process, results in a significantly attenuated drug-induced behavioral sensitization (Tsukamoto et al., 2001). Clearly, additional studies are required to more directly elucidate the functional significance of NAc LTD as it relates to addiction. For example, drug-induced behavioral modification of animals in which NAc LTD is prevented (e.g. by PP1 peptide, (Morishita et al., 2001), or in which excitatory synaptic strength is otherwise decreased would prove particularly illuminating.

Other Brain Regions

The prefrontal cortex, which provides the major excitatory inputs to the brain reward pathway, functions to mediate working memory, impulsive behavior and reward-related learning (Jentsch and Taylor 1999). There have been no studies directly addressing the effect of repeated administration of psychostimulants on excitatory synaptic transmission within the PFC although one study shows that the PFC neurons in amphetamine-pretreated rats exhibited enhanced glutamate responsiveness to glutamate (Peterson et al., 2000), implying that a possible LTP like process may occur in the PFC following drug exposure. On the other hand, it has been consistently demonstrated that cocaine exposure increases the intrinsic membrane excitability of PFC pyramidal neurons by affecting ion channel activity (Dong et al., 2005; Nasif et al., 2005a; Nasif et al., 2005b). Upregulation of the intrinsic membrane excitability of PFC neurons presumably increases presynaptic neurotransmitter release at the excitatory synapses, a process that may serve as a trigger for drug-induced synaptic plasticity in both the VTA and NAc. In addition, drug-induced LTP in the VTA can presumably increase DA tones in the PFC, which should significantly increase the membrane excitability via D1 receptor-mediated modulation of ionic conductances (Yang and Seamans, 1996; Yang et al., 1996; Dong and White, 2003; Dong et al., 2004). It appears that drug-induced physiological adaptations in the PFC, NAc and VTA comprise a positive feedback loop through which drugs of abuse persistently activate the brain reward pathway.

In the ventral lateral bed nucleus of the stria terminalis excitatory synapses may also generate "LTP" in response to cocaine administration (Dumont et al., 2005). Interestingly this LTP could be induced only when the drug is actively consumed by animals, indicating that the triggering process may require co-activation of other brain regions (e.g. PFC) that participate in goal-directed behaviors. It would be interesting to determine the molecular mechanism of this novel "LTP", as well as the functional and behavioral correlates.

CONCLUSION

"Addictive behavior does not result from repeated drug exposure *per se*, but is a result of learning" (Tzschentke and Schmidt, 2003). The concept that addiction is a maladaptive form of reward/emotion/motivation learning and memory (Kelley, 2004) has been recently more readily embraced by the field. This article has predominately focused on drug-induced synaptic plasticity, an important type of plasticity likely to mediate many forms of learning and memory. However, there are many other forms of neuronal plasticity that are likely to also be important for learning and memory, and may also critically contribute to the addiction process. Thus, drug exposure can also cause persistent changes in the intrinsic membrane properties of neurons within the brain reward pathway, which in turn may contribute to certain addiction-related behaviors, such as the sensitivity to cocaine. While the mechanisms underlying drug-induced structural and functional neuronal adaptations continue to be explored, it should be borne in mind that the link between drug-induced neuronal plasticity and maladaptive reward/emotion memory remains to be firmly established. In large part, a successful outcome will depend upon the continued development of appropriate animal models and behavioral assay with which to assess the affective and emotional states. Indeed, an approach in which our advancing appreciation of the molecular basis of drug-induced neural adaptation is integrated with an understanding of its functional and behavioral correlates remains the best hope for eventually unlocking the secrets to drug addiction.

ACKNOWLEDGEMENTS

We thank Drs. Nick Hastings, Yanhua Huang, and Tung Fong for critical suggestions for the manuscript.

REFERENCES

Badiani A, Robinson TE (2004) Drug-induced neurobehavioral plasticity: the role of environmental context. *Behav. Pharmacol.* 15:327-339.

Bear MF (1996) A synaptic basis for memory storage in the cerebral cortex. *Proc. Natl. Acad. Sci. U S A* 93:13453-13459.

Beique JC, Andrade R (2003) PSD-95 regulates synaptic transmission and plasticity in rat cerebral cortex. *J. Physiol.* 546:859-867.

Beurrier C, Malenka RC (2002) Enhanced inhibition of synaptic transmission by dopamine in the nucleus accumbens during behavioral sensitization to cocaine. *J. Neurosci* 22:5817-5822.

Bonci A, Malenka RC (1999) Properties and plasticity of excitatory synapses on dopaminergic and GABAergic cells in the ventral tegmental area. *J. Neurosci* 19:3723-3730.

Borgland SL, Malenka RC, Bonci A (2004) Acute and chronic cocaine-induced potentiation of synaptic strength in the ventral tegmental area: electrophysiological and behavioral correlates in individual rats. *J. Neurosci.* 24:7482-7490.

Carlezon WA, Jr., Nestler EJ (2002) Elevated levels of GluR1 in the midbrain: a trigger for sensitization to drugs of abuse? *Trends Neurosci* 25:610-615.

Carlezon WA, Jr., Todtenkopf MS, McPhie DL, Pimentel P, Pliakas AM, Stellar JR, Trzcinska M (2001) Repeated exposure to rewarding brain stimulation downregulates GluR1 expression in the ventral tegmental area. *Neuropsychopharmacology* 25:234-241.

Churchill L, Swanson CJ, Urbina M, Kalivas PW (1999) Repeated cocaine alters glutamate receptor subunit levels in the nucleus accumbens and ventral tegmental area of rats that develop behavioral sensitization. *J. Neurochem.* 72:2397-2403.

Colledge M, Snyder EM, Crozier RA, Soderling JA, Jin Y, Langeberg LK, Lu H, Bear MF, Scott JD (2003) Ubiquitination regulates PSD-95 degradation and AMPA receptor surface expression. *Neuron* 40:595-607.

Dong Y, White FJ (2003) Dopamine D1-class receptors selectively modulate a slowly inactivating potassium current in rat medial prefrontal cortex pyramidal neurons. *J. Neurosci* 23:2686-2695.

Dong Y, Saal D, Thomas M, Faust R, Bonci A, Robinson T, Malenka RC (2004) Cocaine-induced potentiation of synaptic strength in dopamine neurons: behavioral correlates in GluRA(-/-) mice. Proc. *Natl. Acad. Sci. U S A* 101:14282-14287.

Dong Y, Nasif FJ, Tsui JJ, Ju WY, Cooper DC, Hu XT, Malenka RC, White FJ (2005) Cocaine-induced plasticity of intrinsic membrane properties in prefrontal cortex pyramidal neurons: adaptations in potassium currents. *J. Neurosc.* 25:936-940.

Dumont EC, Mark GP, Mader S, Williams JT (2005) Self-administration enhances excitatory synaptic transmission in the bed nucleus of the stria terminalis. *Nat. Neurosci* 8:413-414.

El-Husseini Ael D, Schnell E, Dakoji S, Sweeney N, Zhou Q, Prange O, Gauthier-Campbell C, Aguilera-Moreno A, Nicoll RA, Bredt DS (2002) Synaptic strength regulated by palmitate cycling on PSD-95. *Cell* 108:849-863.

Faleiro LJ, Jones S, Kauer JA (2004) Rapid synaptic plasticity of glutamatergic synapses on dopamine neurons in the ventral tegmental area in response to acute amphetamine injection. *Neuropsychopharmacology* 29:2115-2125.

Fitzgerald LW, Ortiz J, Hamedani AG, Nestler EJ (1996) Drugs of abuse and stress increase the expression of GluR1 and NMDAR1 glutamate receptor subunits in the rat ventral tegmental area: common adaptations among cross-sensitizing agents. *J. Neurosci* 16:274-282.

Fourgeaud L, Mato S, Bouchet D, Hemar A, Worley PF, Manzoni OJ (2004) A single in vivo exposure to cocaine abolishes endocannabinoid-mediated long-term depression in the nucleus accumbens. J Neurosci 24:6939-6945.

Gerdeman GL, Ronesi J, Lovinger DM (2002) Postsynaptic endocannabinoid release is critical to long-term depression in the striatum. *Nat. Neurosci* 5:446-451.

Grillner P, Mercuri NB (2002) Intrinsic membrane properties and synaptic inputs regulating the firing activity of the dopamine neurons. *Behav. Brain Res.* 130:149-169.

Gurden H, Takita M, Jay TM (2000) Essential role of D1 but not D2 receptors in the NMDA receptor-dependent long-term potentiation at hippocampal-prefrontal cortex synapses in vivo. *J. Neurosci* 20:RC106.

Gutlerner JL, Penick EC, Snyder EM, Kauer JA (2002) Novel protein kinase A-dependent long-term depression of excitatory synapses. *Neuron* 36: 921-931.

Harris GC, Aston-Jones G (2003) Critical role for ventral tegmental glutamate in preference for a cocaine-conditioned environment. *Neuropsychopharmacology* 28:73-76.

Huang YY, Simpson E, Kellendonk C, Kandel ER (2004) Genetic evidence for the bidirectional modulation of synaptic plasticity in the prefrontal cortex by D1 receptors. *Proc. Natl. Acad. Sci.* U S A 101:3236-3241.

Hyman SE, Malenka RC (2001) Addiction and the brain: the neurobiology of compulsion and its persistence. *Nat. Rev. Neurosci* 2:695-703.

Jones S, Kauer JA (1999) Amphetamine depresses excitatory synaptic transmission via serotonin receptors in the ventral tegmental area. *J. Neurosci* 19:9780-9787.

Kabbaj M, Norton CS, Kollack-Walker S, Watson SJ, Robinson TE, Akil H (2001) Social defeat alters the acquisition of cocaine self-administration in rats: role of individual differences in cocaine-taking behavior. *Psychopharmacology* (Berl) 158:382-387.

Kalivas PW (2004) Glutamate systems in cocaine addiction. *Curr. Opin. Pharmacol* 4:23-29.

Kelley AE (2004) Memory and addiction: shared neural circuitry and molecular mechanisms. *Neuron* 44:161-179.

Kelley AE, Smith-Roe SL, Holahan MR (1997) Response-reinforcement learning is dependent on N-methyl-D-aspartate receptor activation in the nucleus accumbens core. *Proc. Natl. Acad. Sci.* U S A 94:12174-12179.

Kelz MB, Chen J, Carlezon WA, Jr., Whisler K, Gilden L, Beckmann AM, Steffen C, Zhang YJ, Marotti L, Self DW, Tkatch T, Baranauskas G, Surmeier DJ, Neve RL, Duman RS, Picciotto MR, Nestler EJ (1999) Expression of the transcription factor deltaFosB in the brain controls sensitivity to cocaine. *Nature* 401:272-276.

Keys AS, Mark GP, Emre N, Meshul CK (1998) Reduced glutamate immunolabeling in the nucleus accumbens following extended withdrawal from self-administered cocaine. *Synapse* 30:393-401.

Kim HS, Park WK, Jang CG, Oh S (1996) Inhibition by MK-801 of cocaine-induced sensitization, conditioned place preference, and dopamine-receptor supersensitivity in mice. *Brain Res. Bull.* 40:201-207.

Kim JA, Pollak KA, Hjelmstad GO, Fields HL (2004) A single cocaine exposure enhances both opioid reward and aversion through a ventral tegmental area-dependent mechanism. *Proc. Natl. Acad. Sci. U S A* 101:5664-5669.

Kombian SB, Malenka RC (1994) Simultaneous LTP of non-NMDA- and LTD of NMDA-receptor-mediated responses in the nucleus accumbens. *Nature* 368:242-246.

Komiyama NH, Watabe AM, Carlisle HJ, Porter K, Charlesworth P, Monti J, Strathdee DJ, O'Carroll CM, Martin SJ, Morris RG, O'Dell TJ, Grant SG (2002) SynGAP regulates ERK/MAPK signaling, synaptic plasticity, and learning in the complex with postsynaptic density 95 and NMDA receptor. *J. Neurosci* 22:9721-9732.

Law-Tho D, Desce JM, Crepel F (1995) Dopamine favours the emergence of long-term depression versus long-term potentiation in slices of rat prefrontal cortex. *Neurosci Lett.* 188:125-128.

Li Y, Kauer JA (2004) Repeated exposure to amphetamine disrupts dopaminergic modulation of excitatory synaptic plasticity and neurotransmission in nucleus accumbens. *Synapse* 51:1-10.

Li Y, Vartanian AJ, White FJ, Xue CJ, Wolf ME (1997) Effects of the AMPA receptor antagonist NBQX on the development and expression of behavioral sensitization to cocaine and amphetamine. Psychopharmacology (Berl) 134:266-276.

Lu W, Wolf ME (1999) Repeated amphetamine administration alters AMPA receptor subunit expression in rat nucleus accumbens and medial prefrontal cortex. *Synapse* 32:119-131.

Lu W, Monteggia LM, Wolf ME (1999) Withdrawal from repeated amphetamine administration reduces NMDAR1 expression in the rat substantia nigra, nucleus accumbens and medial prefrontal cortex. *Eur. J. Neurosci* 11:3167-3177.

Lu W, Monteggia LM, Wolf ME (2002) Repeated administration of amphetamine or cocaine does not alter AMPA receptor subunit expression in the rat midbrain. *Neuropsychopharmacology* 26:1-13.

Lu W, Chen H, Xue CJ, Wolf ME (1997) Repeated amphetamine administration alters the expression of mRNA for AMPA receptor subunits in rat nucleus accumbens and prefrontal cortex. *Synapse* 26: 269-280.

Malenka RC (2003) Synaptic plasticity and AMPA receptor trafficking. *Ann. N. Y. Acad. Sci.* 1003:1-11.

Malenka RC, Nicoll RA (1999) Long-term potentiation--a decade of progress? *Science* 285:1870-1874.

Malinow R, Malenka RC (2002) AMPA receptor trafficking and synaptic plasticity. *Annu. Rev. Neurosci* 25:103-126.

Marinelli M, Piazza PV (2002) Interaction between glucocorticoid hormones, stress and psychostimulant drugs. *Eur. J. Neurosci* 16:387-394.

Mato S, Chevaleyre V, Robbe D, Pazos A, Castillo PE, Manzoni OJ (2004) A single in-vivo exposure to delta 9THC blocks endocannabinoid-mediated synaptic plasticity. *Nat. Neurosci* 7:585-586.

McFarland K, Kalivas PW (2001) The circuitry mediating cocaine-induced reinstatement of drug-seeking behavior. *J. Neurosci* 21:8655-8663.

Meshul CK, Noguchi K, Emre N, Ellison G (1998) Cocaine-induced changes in glutamate and GABA immunolabeling within rat habenula and nucleus accumbens. *Synapse* 30:211-220.

Migaud M, Charlesworth P, Dempster M, Webster LC, Watabe AM, Makhinson M, He Y, Ramsay MF, Morris RG, Morrison JH, O'Dell TJ, Grant SG (1998) Enhanced long-term potentiation and impaired learning in mice with mutant postsynaptic density-95 protein. *Nature* 396:433-439.

Morishita W, Connor JH, Xia H, Quinlan EM, Shenolikar S, Malenka RC (2001) Regulation of synaptic strength by protein phosphatase 1. *Neuron* 32:1133-1148.

Nakagawa T, Futai K, Lashuel HA, Lo I, Okamoto K, Walz T, Hayashi Y, Sheng M (2004) Quaternary structure, protein dynamics, and synaptic function of SAP97 controlled by L27 domain interactions. *Neuron* 44: 453-467.

Nasif FJ, Hu XT, White FJ (2005a) Repeated cocaine administration increases voltage-sensitive calcium currents in response to membrane depolarization in medial prefrontal cortex pyramidal neurons. *J. Neurosci* 25:3674-3679.

Nasif FJ, Sidiropoulou K, Hu XT, White FJ (2005b) Repeated cocaine administration increases membrane excitability of pyramidal neurons in the rat medial prefrontal cortex. *J. Pharmacol. Exp. Ther.* 312:1305-1313.

Nazarian A, Russo SJ, Festa ED, Kraish M, Quinones-Jenab V (2004) The role of D1 and D2 receptors in the cocaine conditioned place preference of male and female rats. *Brain Res. Bull.* 63:295-299.

Nicola SM, Surmeier J, Malenka RC (2000) Dopaminergic modulation of neuronal excitability in the striatum and nucleus accumbens. *Annu. Rev. Neurosci* 23:185-215.

Ortiz J, Fitzgerald LW, Charlton M, Lane S, Trevisan L, Guitart X, Shoemaker W, Duman RS, Nestler EJ (1995) Biochemical actions of chronic ethanol exposure in the mesolimbic dopamine system. *Synapse* 21:289-298.

Otani S (2003) Prefrontal cortex function, quasi-physiological stimuli, and synaptic plasticity. *J. Physiol. Paris* 97:423-430.

Otani S, Blond O, Desce JM, Crepel F (1998) Dopamine facilitates long-term depression of glutamatergic transmission in rat prefrontal cortex. *Neuroscience* 85:669-676.

Overton PG, Clark D (1997) Burst firing in midbrain dopaminergic neurons. *Brain Res. Brain Res. Rev.* 25:312-334.

Overton PG, Richards CD, Berry MS, Clark D (1999) Long-term potentiation at excitatory amino acid synapses on midbrain dopamine neurons. *Neuroreport.* 10:221-226.

Park WK, Bari AA, Jey AR, Anderson SM, Spealman RD, Rowlett JK, Pierce RC (2002) Cocaine administered into the medial prefrontal cortex reinstates cocaine-seeking behavior by increasing AMPA receptor-mediated glutamate transmission in the nucleus accumbens. *J. Neurosci* 22:2916-2925.

Pennartz CM, Ameerun RF, Groenewegen HJ, Lopes da Silva FH (1993) Synaptic plasticity in an in vitro slice preparation of the rat nucleus accumbens. *Eur. J. Neurosci* 5:107-117.

Peterson JD, Wolf ME, White FJ (2000) Altered responsiveness of medial prefrontal cortex neurons to glutamate and dopamine after withdrawal from repeated amphetamine treatment. *Synapse* 36:342-344.

Piazza PV, Le Moal M (1998) The role of stress in drug self-administration. *Trends Pharmacol. Sci.* 19:67-74.

Robbe D, Bockaert J, Manzoni OJ (2002a) Metabotropic glutamate receptor 2/3-dependent long-term depression in the nucleus accumbens is blocked in morphine withdrawn mice. *Eur. J. Neurosci* 16:2231-2235.

Robbe D, Kopf M, Remaury A, Bockaert J, Manzoni OJ (2002b) Endogenous cannabinoids mediate long-term synaptic depression in the nucleus accumbens. *Proc. Natl. Acad. Sci. U S A* 99:8384-8388.

Robinson TE, Becker JB (1986) Enduring changes in brain and behavior produced by chronic amphetamine administration: a review and evaluation of animal models of amphetamine psychosis. *Brain Res.* 396:157-198.

Robinson TE, Berridge KC (2000) The psychology and neurobiology of addiction: an incentive-sensitization view. *Addiction* 95 Suppl 2:S91-117.

Saal D, Dong Y, Bonci A, Malenka RC (2003) Drugs of abuse and stress trigger a common synaptic adaptation in dopamine neurons. *Neuron* 37:577-582.

Sanchez CJ, Sorg BA (2001) Conditioned fear stimuli reinstate cocaine-induced conditioned place preference. *Brain Res.* 908:86-92.

Sanchez CJ, Bailie TM, Wu WR, Li N, Sorg BA (2003) Manipulation of dopamine d1-like receptor activation in the rat medial prefrontal cortex alters stress- and cocaine-induced reinstatement of conditioned place preference behavior. *Neuroscience* 119:497-505.

Schnell E, Sizemore M, Karimzadegan S, Chen L, Bredt DS, Nicoll RA (2002) Direct interactions between PSD-95 and stargazin control synaptic AMPA receptor number. *Proc. Natl. Acad. Sci. U S A* 99:13902-13907.

Schultz W (2002) Getting formal with dopamine and reward. *Neuron* 36: 241-263.

Shaham Y, Shalev U, Lu L, De Wit H, Stewart J (2003) The reinstatement model of drug relapse: history, methodology and major findings. *Psychopharmacology* (Berl) 168:3-20.

Shi SH, Hayashi Y, Petralia RS, Zaman SH, Wenthold RJ, Svoboda K, Malinow R (1999) Rapid spine delivery and redistribution of AMPA receptors after synaptic NMDA receptor activation. *Science* 284: 1811-1816.

Stein V, House DR, Bredt DS, Nicoll RA (2003) Postsynaptic density-95 mimics and occludes hippocampal long-term potentiation and enhances long-term depression. *J. Neurosci* 23:5503-5506.

Thomas MJ, Malenka RC, Bonci A (2000) Modulation of long-term depression by dopamine in the mesolimbic system. *J. Neurosci* 20: 5581-5586.

Thomas MJ, Beurrier C, Bonci A, Malenka RC (2001) Long-term depression in the nucleus accumbens: a neural correlate of behavioral sensitization to cocaine. *Nat. Neurosci* 4:1217-1223.

Tsukamoto T, Iyo M, Tani K, Sekine Y, Hashimoto K, Ohashi Y, Suzuki K, Iwata Y, Mori N (2001) The effects of FK506, a specific calcineurin inhibitor, on methamphetamine-induced behavioral change and its sensitization in rats. *Psychopharmacology* (Berl) 158:107-113.

Tzschentke TM (2001) Pharmacology and behavioral pharmacology of the mesocortical dopamine system. *Prog. Neurobiol* 63:241-320.

Tzschentke TM, Schmidt WJ (2003) Glutamatergic mechanisms in addiction. *Mol. Psychiatry* 8:373-382.

Ungless MA, Whistler JL, Malenka RC, Bonci A (2001) Single cocaine exposure in vivo induces long-term potentiation in dopamine neurons. *Nature* 411:583-587.

Vanderschuren LJ, Kalivas PW (2000) Alterations in dopaminergic and glutamatergic transmission in the induction and expression of behavioral sensitization: a critical review of preclinical studies. *Psychopharmacology* (Berl) 151:99-120.

White FJ, Hu XT, Zhang XF, Wolf ME (1995) Repeated administration of cocaine or amphetamine alters neuronal responses to glutamate in the mesoaccumbens dopamine system. *J. Pharmacol. Exp. Ther.* 273: 445-454.

Will MJ, Watkins LR, Maier SF (1998) Uncontrollable stress potentiates morphine's rewarding properties. *Pharmacol. Biochem. Behav.* 60: 655-664.

Wise RA, Bozarth MA (1987) A psychomotor stimulant theory of addiction. *Psychol. Rev.* 94:469-492.

Wolf ME (1998) The role of excitatory amino acids in behavioral sensitization to psychomotor stimulants. *Prog. Neurobiol.* 54:679-720.

Wolf ME, Sun X, Mangiavacchi S, Chao SZ (2004) Psychomotor stimulants and neuronal plasticity. *Neuropharmacology* 47 Suppl 1:61-79.

Yang CR, Seamans JK (1996) Dopamine D1 receptor actions in layers V-VI rat prefrontal cortex neurons in vitro: modulation of dendritic-somatic signal integration. *J. Neurosci.* 16:1922-1935.

Yang CR, Seamans JK, Gorelova N (1996) Electrophysiological and morphological properties of layers V-VI principal pyramidal cells in rat prefrontal cortex in vitro. *J. Neurosci* 16:1904-1921.

Yao WD, Gainetdinov RR, Arbuckle MI, Sotnikova TD, Cyr M, Beaulieu JM, Torres GE, Grant SG, Caron MG (2004) Identification of PSD-95 as a regulator of dopamine-mediated synaptic and behavioral plasticity. *Neuron* 41:625-638.

Zamanillo D, Sprengel R, Hvalby O, Jensen V, Burnashev N, Rozov A, Kaiser KM, Koster HJ, Borchardt T, Worley P, Lubke J, Frotscher M, Kelly PH, Sommer B, Andersen P, Seeburg PH, Sakmann B (1999) Importance of AMPA receptors for hippocampal synaptic plasticity but not for spatial learning. *Science* 284:1805-1811.

Zhang XF, Hu XT, White FJ (1998) Whole-cell plasticity in cocaine withdrawal: reduced sodium currents in nucleus accumbens neurons. *J. Neurosci* 18:488-498.

Zhang XF, Cooper DC, White FJ (2002) Repeated cocaine treatment decreases whole-cell calcium current in rat nucleus accumbens neurons. *J. Pharmacol. Exp. Ther.* 301:1119-1125.

In: Synaptic Plasticity
Editors: G. N. McMahon et al.

ISBN: 978-1-62081-004-0
© 2012 Nova Science Publishers, Inc.

Chapter VI

INVOLVEMENT OF ZINC VIA CROSSTALK WITH CALCIUM IN SYNAPTIC PLASTICITY AND NEURODEGENERATION IN THE HIPPOCAMPUS[*]

Atsushi Takeda[†]

Department of Medical Biochemistry, School of Pharmaceutical Sciences, University of Shizuoka, Japan

ABSTRACT

Zinc is released with glutamate from neuron terminals in the hippocampus. Zinc may serve as a negative-feedback factor of presynaptic activity and negatively modulate postsynaptic calcium mobilization. On the other hand, the hippocampus is vulnerable to glutamate excitotoxicity, a final common pathway for numerous pathological processes such as Alzheimer's disease and amyotrophic lateral sclerosis, in addition to stroke/ischemia, temporal lobe epilepsy. The excitotoxicity is linked to the excessive influx of zinc and calcium.

---

[*] A version of this chapter also appears in *Hippocampus: Anatomy, Functions and Neurobiology*, edited by Ambroise Gärtner and Dener Frantz, published by Nova Science Publishers, Inc. It was submitted for appropriate modifications in an effort to encourage wider dissemination of research.
[†] E-mail: takedaa@u-shizuoka-ken.ac.jp.

The crosstalk between zinc and calcium via calcium channels may play a role in both synaptic plasticity and excitotoxicity. This paper summarizes the involvement of zinc in functional and toxic aspects in the hippocampus focused on the crosstalk. The enhanced excitotoxicity in the hippocampus in zinc deficiency is also summarized.

Keywords: Zinc, glutamate, excitotoxicity, hippocampus, calcium, crosstalk, zinc deficiency

1. INTRODUCTION

Zinc is the second most abundant trace element in the body and powerfully influences cell division and differentiation [1, 2]. In microorganisms, plants and animals, over 300 enzymes require zinc for their functions. Zinc has three functions in zinc enzymes: catalytic, coactive (or cocatalytic) and structural [3]. In the brain, zinc turnover is strictly regulated via the brain-barrier system [4, 5]. Averaged intracellular zinc concentration is estimated to be approximately 150 µM, judging from zinc concentration in the total brain, while extracellular zinc concentration is estimated to be approximately 0.15−1 µM, judging from zinc concentration in the cerebrospinal fluid and extracellular zinc concentration measured by in vivo microdialysis. Zinc serves as an intracellular and an extracellular signal factor in synaptic neurotransmission; approximately 90 % of the total brain zinc forms zinc metalloproteins. The rest exists in the presynaptic vesicles and is histochemically reactive (as revealed by Timm's sulfide-silver staining method) [6, 7].

Zinc concentration is relatively high in the hippocampus in the brain [8] and the action of zinc is closely linked to functions and pathological processes [9]. There is a large number of evidence on zinc-containing glutamatergic neurons that sequester zinc in the presynaptic vesicles and release it in a calcium- and impulse-dependent manner [7, 10]. Zinc concentration in the presynaptic vesicles is the highest in the giant boutons of hippocampal mossy fibers and is estimated to be approximately 300 µM there [11]. All giant boutons of mossy fibers contain zinc in the presynaptic vesicles, while approximately 45% of Schaffer collateral boutons is zinc-positive [12]. Vesicular zinc may serve as an endogenous neuromodulator of several important receptors including the α-amino-3-hydroxy-5-methyl-4-isoxazolepropionic acid (AMPA)/kainate receptor, N-methyl-D-aspartate (NMDA) and γ-amino butyric acid (GABA) receptors [13-15]. However, the extracellular concentration of zinc reached after the release is a matter of debate. Estimates after tetanic stimulation range between 10 and 100 µM [16, 17], even up to 300 µM under extreme conditions [18]. Excess of extracellular zinc become neurotoxic via the translocation of zinc to postsynaptic neurons [19-23].

This paper summarizes zinc action via crosstalk between zinc and calcium in both functional and pathological aspects and also enhanced glutamate excitotoxicity in zinc deficiency.

2. ZINC TRANSPORT INTO THE BRAIN

Zinc-binding affinity for ligands in the plasma is important to understand the mechanism of zinc transport into the brain through the brain barrier system (Figure 1) [4]. Plasma zinc (approximately 15 µM) is partitioned between high molecular–weight and low molecular–weight fractions. The former is a protein–bound form (98 %) and the latter is a low molecular–weight ligand–bound form (1–2 %) and free zinc (Zn^{2+}), which is estimated to be as low as 10^{-9}–10^{-10} M.

The largest component of exchangeable zinc in the plasma is albumin. A brain autoradiogram with ^{65}Zn in the Nagase analbuminemic rat, which has a genetic mutation affecting albumin mRNA processing and lacks plasma albumin, demonstrated that ^{65}Zn distribution in the brain is similar to that in normal rats and that albumin is not essential for zinc transport into the brain [24].

However, plasma albumin appears to participate in zinc transport as a large pool of exchangeable zinc in normal animals. Zinc is also known to bind to other plasma proteins such as transferrin and $α_2$–macroglobulin. Although zinc firmly binds to $α_2$-macroglobulin, its functional significance is unknown.

The next largest component of exchangeable zinc in the plasma is amino acids, *i.e.*, histidine and cysteine. Aiken *et al.* reported that the ratio of ^{65}Zn concentration in the brain, as well as in other tissues, to plasma ^{65}Zn concentration is enhanced by L-histidine infusion [25]. Brain distribution of ^{65}Zn-His is consistent with the data of an L-histidine infusion experiment [26]. It is possible that L-histidine is involved in zinc transport into the brain parenchyma through the brain barrier system [27]. A rat brain peptide/histidine transporter (PHT1) has been cloned [28]. PHT1 mRNA is intensely expressed in the choroid plexus. However, it is unknown whether histidine-bound forms actually pass across the plasma membranes of the choroidal epithelial cells (and brain capillary endothelial cells). On the other hand, DMT1, a divalent metal transporter, is expressed in brain capillary endothelial cells and choroidal epithelial cells [29]. Alternatively, it is possible that histidine serves to transfer zinc to DMT1. Other zinc transporters, e.g., hZIP (ZRT1, IRT1-like protein), are also candidates for zinc transport across the brain barrier system [30].

Zinc is transported into the brain across the blood-CSF barrier, in addition to the blood-brain barrier, the main supply path of zinc (Figure 1); the choroid plexus might participate in slow supply of zinc to the brain. ^{65}Zn was highly distributed in the choroid plexus of mice and rats 1 h after intravenous injection of ^{65}ZnCl$_2$ and then distributed in the brain parenchyma with a decrease in choroidal ^{65}Zn [8]. The maximum concentrations of ^{65}Zn in the rat brain were observed 6–10 days after the injection [31]. In the brain, ^{65}Zn was concentrated in the hippocampus, especially the hippocampal CA3 and dentate gyrus, and also in the amygdala, especially the amygdalopiriform transition and the amygdalo-hippocampal transition areas.

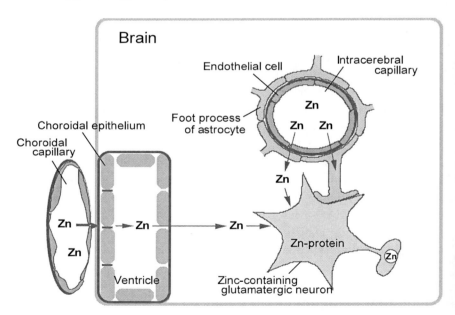

Figure 1. Zinc transport into the brain via the brain barrier system. Zinc bound to albumin and amino acids, i.e., histidine and cysteine, serves as the exchangeable zinc pool in the plasma. Zinc is transported into the brain through the blood-brain and the blood-CSF barriers.

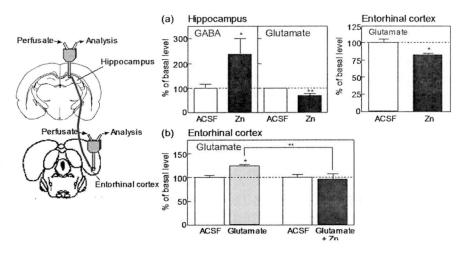

Figure 2. Zinc-dependent response of hippocampal CA1-entorhinal cortex connection. Position of microdialysis probes in the hippocampal CA1 and the entorhinal cortex is shown in the brain maps. a, When the hippocampal CA1 was perfused with ACSF for 60 min and then with 50 μM ZnCl$_2$ in ACSF for 30 min, the entorhinal cortex was perfused with ACSF alone. Each bar and line represent the mean ± s.e.m. The asterisks indicate significant differences (*, $p<0.05$; **, $p<0.01$) from the basal level (ACSF). b, When the hippocampal CA1 was perfused with ACSF for 60 min and then with 50 μM glutamate in ACSF or 50 μM glutamate + 50 μM ZnCl$_2$ in ACSF for 30 min, the entorhinal cortex was perfused with ACSF alone. Each bar and line represents the mean ± s.e.m. The asterisks indicate significant differences (*, $p<0.05$; **, $p<0.01$) from ACSF or glutamate group.

Zinc concentration in the CSF is approximately 0.15 μM. To study zinc uptake by the brain parenchyma cells *via* the CSF, ^{65}ZnCl$_2$ and ^{65}Zn-His were injected intracerebroventricularly in rats [32, 33]. ^{65}Zn was distributed in the brain parenchyma, *i.e.*, the hippocampus and hypothalamus, after intracerebroventricular injection of ^{65}ZnCl$_2$, while the radioactivity from ^{65}Zn-His was distributed extensively in the brain compared with that from ^{65}ZnCl$_2$. PHT1 mRNA is widely expressed in the brain [28]. Especially intense hybridization signals are found in the hippocampus, cerebellum, and pontine nucleus. It is possible that PHT1 is involved in zinc uptake in neurons and glial cells. On the other hand, the finding that histidine decreases ^{65}Zn uptake in the synaptosomal preparation suggests that histidine does not participate in a carrier-mediated uptake in neuron terminals [34]. Therefore, the mechanism of zinc uptake by neurons and glial cells remains to be clarified. On the other hand, calcium channels are involved in zinc uptake in excitation (depolarization) of zinc-containing glutamatergic neurons as described later (Figure 6) [35,36]; zinc influx via calcium channels is linked to not only the modulation of zinc-containing glutamatergic neuron activity but also neurodegeneration.

Zinc turnover in the brain is very slow in contrast to zinc dynamics in the synaptic activity. The half-time for elimination of ^{65}Zn from the rat brain is in the range of 16–43 days; the longest is observed in the amygdala, followed by those in the piriform cortex and perirhinal cortex [31].

3. DIFFERENTIAL ACTION OF EXTRACELLULAR ZINC IN EXTRACELLULAR NEUROTRANSMITTER CONCENTRATIONS

Zinc taken up by neurons is transported anterogradely and retrogradely *via* the axonal transport system [37,38]. In zinc-containing glutamatergic neurons, the zinc may be transported into synaptic vesicles (Figure 1). Zinc sequestered in the synaptic vesicles is released with glutamate into the synaptic cleft [7]. However, the role of vesicular zinc is poorly understood. To examine the action of extracellular zinc in extracellular glutamate concentration, *in vivo* microdialysis experiments were carried out in the rat hippocampus. In the hippocampal CA3 region innervated by mossy fibers of dentate granule cells, glutamate concentration in the extracellular fluid was decreased by perfusion with 10–300 μM ZnCl$_2$, while increased by perfusion with 1 mM CaEDTA, a membrane-impermeable zinc chelator, suggesting that endogenous zinc released into the synaptic cleft attenuates glutamate release in the CA3 region [39]. On the other hand, GABA concentration in the extracellular fluid was increased by perfusion with zinc, while decreased by perfusion with CaEDTA. Extracellular zinc may differentially act on glutamatergic and GABAergic neurotransmitter systems.

The hippocampal CA1 is connected with CA3 pyramidal cells *via* Schaffer collaterals (Figure 3). Extracellular glutamate concentration was also decreased by perfusion with zinc in the CA1 region. Thus, zinc action in the postsynaptic response (glutamate release) was examined by using the CA1–entorhinal connection (Figure 2) [40]. Perfusion of the CA1 with 1 μM tetrodotoxin, a sodium channel blocker, significantly decreased extracellular glutamate concentration in the entorhinal cortex, while perfusion of the CA1 with 50 μM glutamate significantly increased it, indicating that the response of postsynaptic CA1 pyramidal cells can be monitored by the level of glutamate released from the neuron terminals in the entorhinal cortex. When the CA1 region was perfused with 50 µM $ZnCl_2$, extracellular glutamate concentration was decreased not only in the CA1 but also in the entorhinal cortex (Figure 2a). Furthermore, the increase in extracellular glutamate concentration in the entorhinal cortex during perfusion of the CA1 with 50 µM glutamate was completely suppressed by addition of 50 µM $ZnCl_2$ to the CA1 (Figure 2b). Zinc could potentiate AMPA/kainate receptors, a subtype of glutamate receptors, on CA1 pyramidal cells [41].

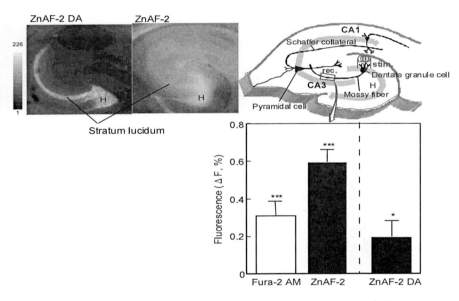

Figure 3. Zinc dynamics in intracellular and extracellular compartments in the hippocampus. ZnAF-2 DA and ZnAF-2 was applied to rat hippocampal slices to image intracellular and extracellular zinc, respectively. The fluorescent signal was imaged with an Argus-50/CA. H, hilus. In another experiment, hippocampal slices were double-stained with Fura-2 AM and ZnAF-2. Hippocampal slices were also stained with ZnAF-2 DA. Tetanic stimuli at 100 Hz for 1 s were delivered to the dentate granule cell layer and the fluorescent signals were monitored with a confocal laser-scanning microscopic system LSM 510 at the rate of 1 Hz through a 10 × objective. Region of interest was set in the stratum lucidum. The data represent the increment (%) of fluorescent signal during the stimulation (1 s) to the basal fluorescent signal just before the stimulation (the mean of 3 s). Each bar and line represents the mean ± S.E.M. *, $p<0.05$, **, $p<0.001$, vs. the basal level before the stimulation.

However, in addition to the attenuation of glutamate release from presynaptic neurons, the inhibition of NMDA receptors on the CA1 pyramidal cells and the enhancement of GABA release from interneurons, which are both mediated by zinc, appear to attenuate the above potentiation, resulting in the attenuation of glutamate release from the postsynaptic neuron terminals.

4. ZINC DYNAMICS ALONG WITH NEURONAL ACTIVITY

In the brain extracellular fluid, zinc seems to consist of two forms mainly. One is the form bound to low molecular weight ligands such as amino acids and another is free zinc (Zn^{2+}) [4]. Free zinc concentration in the extracellular fluid is estimated to be approximately 20 nM [42]. ZnAF-2, a membrane-impermeable zinc indicator, has a low K_d value of 2.7 nM for zinc and its fluorescence is minimally changed in the presence of calcium, magnesium, cadmium, nickel or other heavy metals [43,44]. ZnAF-2 also has no apparent toxicity to living cells. To observe zinc dynamics during excitation of mossy fiber synapses, intracellular zinc in hippocampal slices was stained with membrane-permeable ZnAF-2 DA, diacetylated form of ZnAF-2. ZnAF-2 DA taken up by cells is hydrolyzed to ZnAF-2, which cannot permeate the cell membrane (Figure 3). Intracellular ZnAF-2 signal was highly detected in the dentate hilus and stratum lucidum, in which mossy fibers exist.

On the other hand, when ZnAF-2 was added to hippocampal slices, extracellular ZnAF-2 signal was immediately detected in the dentate hilus and stratum lucidum. The fluorescent signal was also detected around their regions.

When tetanic stimuli at 100 Hz for 1 s were delivered to the dentate granule cell layer, both extracellular and intracellular ZnAF-2 signals were increased with intracellular calcium (Fura-2) signal in the stratum lucidum during the stimulation (Figure 3) [45]. It is possible that the increase in intracellular ZnAF-2 signal is due to the binding of cytosolic ZnAF-2 to zinc retaken up after the release and that the increment in cytosolic signal is more than the decrement in vesicular signal. This possibility is supported by the data that the increase in intracellular ZnAF-2 signal in mossy fiber terminals during the tetanic stimulation was significantly decreased in the presence of 1 mM CaEDTA (Figure 4) [45]. Zinc released from mossy fiber terminals during tetanic stimulation may be immediately retaken up by the mossy fibers, probably via calcium channels such as VDCC, and also taken up into postsynaptic CA3 neurons.

Involvement of Zinc via Crosstalk with Calcium ...

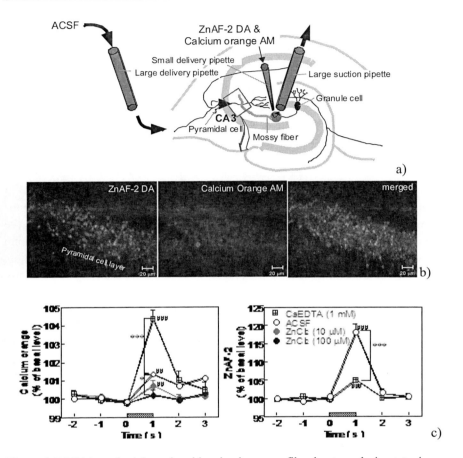

Figure 4. Inhibition of calcium signal by zinc in mossy fiber boutons during tetanic stimulation. a, Schematic illustration of the procedure. The stratum lucidum was regionally perfused with ZnAF-2 DA and calcium orange AM for mossy fiber terminal labeling. The red square was observed as shown in b. b, Giant boutons of mossy fibers were double-labeled with calcium orange and ZnAF-2 as shown in a merged image. c, Tetanic stimuli at 100 Hz for 1 s were delivered to the dentate granule cell layer in ACSF or reagents in ACSF. The fluorescent signals were monitored with a confocal laser-scanning microscopic system LSM 510 at the rate of 1 Hz through a 20 □ objective. Region of interest (around 5 □m in diameter) was set in giant boutons of mossy fibers double-labeled with calcium orange and ZnAF-2. The data represent the ratio (%) of each fluorescent signal (1 s) to the basal fluorescent signal (the mean of 3 s) just before the stimulation. Each point and line represents the mean ± S.E.M. The shaded bar indicates the period of the stimulation. *, $p<0.05$, **, $p<0.001$, vs. ACSF group; **, $p<0.01$, ***, $p<0.001$, vs. the basal level (the mean of 3 points just before the stimulation).

5. ZINC ACTION VIA CROSSTALK BETWEEN ZINC AND CALCIUM IN FUNCTIONAL ASPECT

Neural circuits of the zinc-containing glutamatergic neurons are considered to be associated with the episodic memory function and are important for behavior, emotional expression and cognitive-mnemonic operations [4]. Lu et al. [46] demonstrated that endogenous zinc is required for the induction of long-term potentiation (LTP) in hippocampal mossy fiber synapses. Li et al. [47] demonstrated that the induction of LTP in hippocampal mossy fiber synapses requires translocation of synaptically released zinc. On the other hand, the impairment of spatial learning, memory or sensorimotor function was not observed in zinc transporter-3-null mice, which lack the histochemically reactive zinc in synaptic vesicles [48,49]. There is also some evidence that zinc has no role in the CA3 mossy fiber LTP [16,50]. Thus, clarifying the physiological significance of vesicular zinc in synaptic plasticity is important to understand the hippocampal function.

The presynaptic action of zinc released from mossy fibers during tetanic stimulation was examined by using rat hippocampal slices (Figure 4). In mossy fiber terminals preferentially double-stained with zinc and calcium indicators, the increase in calcium orange signal during delivery of tetanic stimuli (100 Hz, 1 s) to the dentate granule cell layer is enhanced in the presence of 1 mM CaEDTA and attenuated in the presence of 100 µM zinc [45]. It is likely that zinc released from mossy fiber terminals suppresses the increase in calcium signal (Ca^{2+}) in the presynaptic terminals induced by tetanic stimulation, followed by inhibitory modulation of the presynaptic activity (Figure 5). Presynaptic calcium influx through voltage-dependent calcium cannel (VDCC) triggers vesicular exocytosis. FM4-64, a fluorescent indicator of synaptic vesicle recycling, is taken up into presynaptic vesicles in an activity-dependent manner. Subsequent rounds of exocytosis arising from depolarization lead to the release of the dye from the presynaptic terminals (destaining) [51, 52].

When tetanic stimuli at 10 Hz for 180 s, which induce mossy fiber LTP, are delivered to the dentate granule cell layer, the decrease in FM4-64 signal is enhanced by addition of 1 mM CaEDTA and suppressed by addition of 100 µM zinc [45]. Zinc released from mossy fiber terminals during tetanic stimulation may suppress vesicular exocytosis, via inhibitory modulation of presynaptic calcium mobilization (Figure 5).

The hippocampal mossy fiber LTP is expressed by presynaptic mechanisms leading to persistent enhancement of neurotransmitter release. The induction of mossy fiber LTP is critically dependent on the increase in presynaptic calcium induced by stimulation of depolarization [53-55], which activates the calcium-calmodulin-sensitive adenyl cyclase I [56]. Mossy fiber zinc might be involved in the presynaptic mechanism leading to the LTP and be a negative neuromodulator against the presynaptic mechanism. It is possible that the release from mossy fibers leads to cross talk between extracellular free zinc and calcium via calcium channels such as VDCC, which is inhibited by zinc [57]. In an experiment using synaptosomal fraction of rat hippocampal CA3, on the other hand, zinc inhibits glutamate release via activation of presynaptic ATP-dependent potassium (K_{ATP}) channel [58]. Low micromolar concentrations of zinc inhibit cAMP signaling via inhibition of adenyl cyclase in N18TG2 neuroblastoma cells [59]. The IC_{50} of zinc against recombinant adenyl cyclase I is 1.4 µM. It is also possible that zinc taken up into the mossy fibers suppresses the cAMP-PKA signaling pathway via inhibition of adenyl cyclase I in mossy fiber boutons.

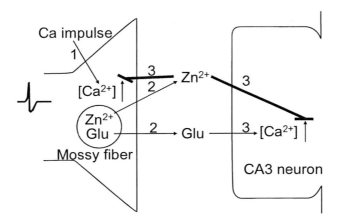

Figure 5. Negative zinc action against calcium mobilization in mossy fiber excitation. When the action potential is delivered to mossy fibers, calcium influx occurs via voltage-dependent calcium channel (VDCC) and Ca2+ concentration increases in the terminals (1), followed by exocytosis (2). Zinc released from mossy fiber boutons may negatively modulate the presynaptic activity via suppression of the increase in Ca2+ concentration (3). The negative modulation of the presynaptic activity by zinc leads to suppression of postsynaptic calcium mobilization. Zinc also negatively modulates the increase in Ca2+ concentration in postsynaptic CA3 neurons (3).

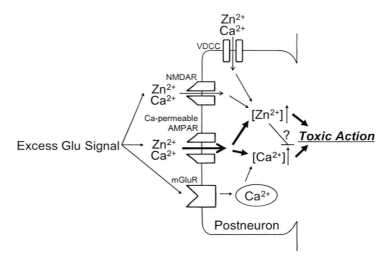

Figure 6. Zinc action in excessive excitation of mossy fibers. Excess of extracellular glutamate triggers excessive influx of zinc and calcium into postsynaptic CA3 neurons via ionotropic glutamate receptors and VDCC, followed by neurodegeneration. Calcium-permeable AMPA/kainite receptors play an important role in neurodegenerative processes. Extracellular zinc suppresses calcium mobilization into postsynaptic CA3 neurons via blockade of NMDA receptors and VDCC. The increase in intracellular zinc may suppress calcium release from internal stores, although it is harmful to postsynaptic CA3 neurons.

To examine zinc uptake by CA3 pyramidal cells and its significance, zinc uptake was checked in the CA3 pyramidal cell layer stained with ZnAF-2DA after tetanic stimulation to the dentate granule cell layer. The increase in intracellular ZnAF-2 signal induced by tetanic stimulation was completely inhibited in the presence of CNQX, an AMPA/kainate receptor antagonist [35]. These results suggest that zinc released from mossy fibers is taken up into CA3 pyramidal cells via activation of AMPA/kainate receptors. Activation of AMPA/kainate receptors provides the membrane depolarization and activates NMDA receptors and VDCC. Therefore, it is likely that calcium channels such as NMDA receptors and VDCC, in addition to calcium-permeable AMPA/kainate (GluR2-lacking) receptors, are involved in zinc uptake into CA3 pyramidal cells after mossy fiber excitation (Figure 6) [22].

Mossy fiber activity evokes intracellular calcium mobilization via group I metabotropic glutamate receptors in CA3 pyramidal cells, in addition to calcium influx via NMDA receptors and VDCC, which is inhibited by zinc (Figure 6) [60]. Group I metabotropic glutamate receptors are coupled to phospholipase C and their activation evokes calcium release from internal stores via IP$_3$ [61,62]; tADA stimulates phosphoinositide hydrolysis and calcium release from internal stores [60,63]. It is possible that the increase in free zinc concentration in CA3 pyramidal cells by mossy fiber activity influence calcium mobilization via group I metabotropic glutamate receptors. Group I metabotropic glutamate receptor activation is associated with memory formation. tADA facilitates maintenance of LTP in the dentate gyrus in vivo and memory formation in the spatial alteration task [64,65]. On the other hand, group I metabotropic glutamate receptor activation is also associated with neurotoxic effects of glutamate in post-ischemic neuronal damage and epileptiform activity [61,62]. Because group I metabotropic glutamate receptor activation is involved in both functional and toxic aspects, it seems to be important to understand the effect of free zinc levels on intracellular calcium mobilization. Cytosolic concentration of basal free zinc is estimated to be subnanomlar [66]. The action of free zinc levels in CA3 pyramidal cells after group I metabotropic glutamate receptor activation was examined by regional delivery of tADA to the stratum lucidum after blockade of AMPA/kainate receptor-mediated calcium and zinc influx [35]. Intracellular calcium orange signal in the CA3 pyramidal cell layer was increased by tADA, suggesting that calcium release from internal stores is induced by group I metabotropic glutamate receptor activation in CA3 pyramidal cells (Figure 6). Furthermore, pyrithione was used to manipulate intracellular free zinc concentration [35]. The perfusion with 50 μM pyrithione decreased basal ZnAF-2 signal in the CA3 pyramidal cell layer without affecting basal calcium orange signal. The increase in calcium orange signal in the CA3 pyramidal cell layer by tADA was enhanced in the presence of 50 μM pyrithione. These results suggest that calcium mobilization via group I metabotropic glutamate receptor pathway is facilitated by the decrease in free zinc concentration in CA3 pyramidal cells. The perfusion with 50 μM pyrithione and 100 μM zinc increased basal ZnAF-2 signal in the CA3 pyramidal cell layer and deceased basal calcium orange signal, suggesting that basal free calcium concentration is decreased by the increase in free zinc concentration in CA3 pyramidal cells. The increase in calcium orange signal by tADA was blocked in the presence of 50 μM pyrithione and 100 μM zinc, suggesting that calcium mobilization via group I metabotropic glutamate receptor pathway is blocked by the increase in free zinc concentration in CA3 pyramidal cells (Figure 5 and 6). Therefore, zinc influx via AMPA/kainate receptor activation may negatively modulate calcium mobilization via group I metabotropic glutamate receptor pathway in CA3 pyramidal cells after mossy fiber excitation. It is possible that the negative modulation by zinc is linked to not only synaptic plasticity such as LTP and long-term depression (LTD) but also a neuroprotective function [61]; activation of group I metabotropic glutamate receptors amplifies NMDA-mediated neuronal toxicity and blockade of them is neuroprotective against NMDA-mediated damage. However, excessive zinc influx via AMPA/kainate receptor activation may be neurotoxic in postsynaptic neurons [19-23], even if the zinc negatively modulates intracellular calcium mobilization (Figure 5 and 6).

6. ZINC ACTION VIA CROSSTALK BETWEEN ZINC AND CALCIUM IN THE PATHOLOGICAL ASPECT

In global ischemia, CA1 pyramidal neurons degenerate, whereas CA3 pyramidal neurons remain intact [67-68]. Excess of extracellular glutamate is known as excitotoxicity. It is possible that mossy fiber zinc serves protectively against glutamate excitotoxicity elicited by excessive excitation of dentate granule cells, although excess of extracellular zinc is also harmful because of the translocation to the postneuron as described above. The response of hippocampal mossy fiber zinc to excessive glutamate release was examined by regional delivery of 1 mM glutamate to the stratum lucidum [69]. Extracelluar zinc signal was markedly increased in the stratum lucidum and intracellular calcium signal was persistently increased in the CA3 pyramidal cell layer. These results suggest that the excessive delivery of glutamate leads to the release of zinc and glutamate from mossy fibers and excites mossy fiber synapses. Presynaptic kainate receptors is involved in glutamate release [70]. Excessive delivery of glutamate activates presynaptic kainate receptors, followed by the release of zinc and glutamate from mossy fibers. Excessive delivery of glutamate may also facilitate glutamate release from astrocyres via activation of AMPA/kainate receptors [71].

The persistent increase in calcium signal in the CA3 pyramidal cell layer during stimulation with glutamate was significantly attenuated in the presence of 100 µM zinc, while significantly enhanced in the presence of 1 mM CaEDTA [69]. These results suggest that zinc released from mossy fibers attenuates the increase in intracellular calcium signal in mossy fiber synapses and postsynaptic CA3 neurons after excessive inputs to dentate granular cells (Figure 5). The blockade of calcium influx via NMDA receptors and VDCC by zinc may be involved in attenuating the increase in intracellular calcium.

Furthermore, zinc may inhibit intracellular calcium mobilization via activation of group I metabotropic glutamate receptors as described above (Figure 6). An enhanced GABA release from interneurons by zinc might be also involved in attenuating the increase in calcium signal in mossy fibers and postsynaptic CA3 neurons [39]. Extracelullar and intracellular action of zinc seems to be linked to negative modulation of the increase in intracellular calcium in mossy fiber synapses (Figure 5). Therefore, excessive zinc release from mossy fibers is involved in both functional and toxic aspects.

The role of zinc in excitation of Schaffer collateral-CA1 pyramidal cell synapses was examined by using hippocampal slices stained with ZnAF-2 and ZnAF-2DA [36]. Extracellular and intracellular ZnAF-2 signals were increased in the stratum radiatum of the CA1, in which Schaffer collateral synapses exist, during tetanic stimulation (200 Hz, 1 s). Both the increases were completely blocked in the presence of 1 mM CaEDAT, suggesting that 1 mM CaEDTA is effective to chelate zinc released from Schaffer collaterals. The increase in intracellular fura-2 signal in the stratum radiatum of the CA1 during delivery of tetanic stimuli at 100 Hz for 1 s to the Schaffer collaterals is significantly enhanced in the presence of CaEDTA [72], suggesting that zinc released from Schaffer collaterals negatively modulates presynaptic and/or postsynaptic calcium signaling in the CA1. The presynaptic action of Schaffer collateral zinc was examined by using FM4-64 [36]. The decrease in FM4-64 signal during tetanic stimulation (10 Hz, 180 s) was enhanced in the stratum radiatum of the CA1 (Schaffer collaterals) in the presence of 1 mM CaEDTA, while suppressed in the presence of 5 μM $ZnCl_2$, suggesting that zinc released from Schaffer collaterals suppresses presynaptic activity during tetanic stimulation. When Schaffer collateral synapses were regionally stimulated with 1 mM glutamate, calcium orange signal was increased in the CA1 pyramidal cell layer. This increase was enhanced in the presence of 1 mM CaEDTA and attenuated in the presence of 10 μM $ZnCl_2$. These results suggest that zinc attenuates excitation of Schaffer collateral synapses elicited with glutamate via suppression of presynaptic activity and inhibition of postsynaptic NMDA receptors. Schaffer collateral zinc may also negatively modulate intracellular calcium signal in excessive excitation of Schaffer collateral synapses.

7. ZINC AND EPILEPSY

Zinc homeostasis in the brain is closely associated with epileptic seizures [9]; zinc concentration in the brain is decreased by epileptic seizures [73]. Kainate is an agonist of glutamate receptor subtypes and kainate-challenged mice and rats are experimental models of human temporal lobe epilepsy. They have been used to understand brain zinc movement in epileptic seizures. Zinc concentration in the hippocampus is significantly decreased in kainate-challenged mice [73]. A selective loss of Timm's stain is observed in the hippocampal mossy fibers after electrical stimulation of the perforant path, which evokes hippocampal granule spikes and epileptiform discharges [74,75]. Extracellular concentrations of zinc and glutamate are significantly increased in the hippocampus of young rats challenged with kainate [76]. The attenuation of Timm's stain is due to excessive excitation of zinc-containing glutamatergic neurons, followed by the translocation of zinc to postsynaptic neurons and neurodegeneration. Neuronal loss is observed in the CA1, CA2 and CA3 pyramidal cell layers after challenge with kainite [77] and seems to be linked to the loss of zinc from the hippocampus [73].

8. ZINC AND NOVELTY STRESS

Acute stress enhances hypothalamo-pituitary-adrenocortical (HPA) axis activity. Painful physical stress such as electro footshocks, restraint, forced swimming and tail pinch enhances the HPA axis activity, while a novel environment that an animal has not previously experienced can also influence the HPA axis activity [78,79]. An animal suddenly placed in a novel environment for a specified period shows a complex behavior for exploratory activity [80,81]. This placement is a novelty stress and is regarded as painless psychological stress. Exploratory activity involves several processes, including arousal, attention and locomotor activity and is associated with anxiety, fear and stress [82]. An extensive neuronal activity takes place in the hippocampus during exploratory behavior [83]. The hippocampal function is linked with the HPA axis activity and is involved in stress response [84].

To analyze the response of extracellular zinc in the hippocampus against novelty stress, rats were placed for 50 min in a novel environment once a day for 8 days [85]. Extracellular glutamate in the hippocampus was increased during exploratory behavior on day 1, whereas extracellular zinc was decreased. The same phenomenon was observed during exploratory behavior on day 2 and extracellular zinc returned to the basal level during exploratory behavior on day 8. To examine the significance of the decrease in extracellular zinc in exploratory activity, exploratory behavior was observed under perfusion with 1 mM CaEDTA. Locomotor activity in the novel environment was decreased by perfusion with CaEDTA. The decrease in extracellular zinc and the increase in extracellular glutamate in exploratory period were abolished by perfusion with CaEDTA. These results suggest that zinc uptake by hippocampal cells is linked with exploratory activity and required for the activation of glutamatergic neurotransmitter system. The zinc uptake may be involved in the response in painless psychological stress or the cognitive processes.

9. ENHANCED GLUTAMATE EXCITOTOXICITY IN ZINC DEFICIENCY

Approximately 50% of the world population does not get adequate zinc [86]. Dietary zinc deficiency not only retards the growth of humans and animals, but also affects brain maturation [87,88]. Inadequate dietary zinc causes changes in behavior such as reduced activity and responsiveness. Periods of rapid growth such as pregnancy and infancy are particularly susceptible to dietary zinc deficiency.

Dietary zinc deficiency causes a decrease in the plasma zinc concentration [89], probably in the exchangeable zinc pool, followed by a decrease in the zinc concentration in the liver and femur. On the other hand, several researchers failed to find any change in brain zinc concentration in dietary zinc deficiency [9, 87]. Although zinc concentration in the hippocampus was not decreased after 4-week zinc deprivation, hippocampal extracellular zinc and histochemically reactive zinc detected by Timm's staining were decreased in young rats and mice fed a zinc-deficient diet for 4 weeks [76, 90]. Furthermore, zinc concentration in the hippocampus was significantly decreased after 12-week zinc deprivation [91]. The hippocampus is responsive to dietary zinc deficiency and vesicular zinc seems to be more responsive to dietary zinc deficiency than zinc metalloproteins.

Alteration of zinc homeostasis in the brain influences the etiology and manifestation of epileptic seizures [92-95]. Susceptibility to kainate-induced seizures was enhanced in mice and rats fed a zinc-deficient diet for 4 weeks

[76,96]. Enhanced release of glutamate associated with a decrease in GABA concentration in the hippocampus is a possible mechanism for the enhanced seizure susceptibility in zinc deficiency. Neuronal loss and TUNEL-positive cells are more observed in the CA1, CA2 and CA3 pyramidal cell layers of zinc-deficient group than those of the control group after challenge with kainite [77]; kainate-induced excitotoxcity is enhanced by zinc deficiency (Figure 7).

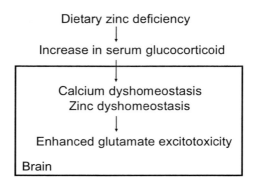

Figure 7. Enhanced glutamate excitotoxicity in the hippocampus in zinc deficiency. Zinc deficiency activates the HPA axis, followed by the increase in serum corticosterone, and increases the basal levels of intracellular Ca2+ in the hippocampus prior to the decrease in extracellular zinc. Intracellular calcium dyshomeostasis, in addition to zinc dyshomeostasis, may be linked to the enhanced glutamate excitotoxicity in the hippocampus in zinc deficiency.

Glutamate excitotoxicity is a final common pathway for numerous pathological processes such as Alzheimer's disease and amyotrophic lateral sclerosis, in addition to stroke/ischemia, temporal lobe epilepsy [97,98]. It is likely that pathological processes associated with glutamate excitotoxicity are aggravated by zinc deficiency. Therefore, adequate zinc supply to the brain is important for prevention of neurological diseases.

10. ACTIVATION OF HPA AXIS IN EARLY ZINC DEFICIENCY

Dietary zinc deficiency causes anorexia, followed by weight loss and growth retardation [99-101]. It is possible that the stress of severe food restriction leads to the increase in serum corticosterone concentration via activation of the HPA axis; serum corticosterone concentration is significantly increased in young rats after 2-week zinc deprivation (Figure 7) [102]. The activation of HPA axis occurs prior to the decrease in extracellular zinc and histochemically reactive zinc in the hippocampus in zinc deficiency. Behavioral abnormality in the open-field test and the increase in anxiety-like behavior are observed in young rats after 2-week zinc deprivation, suggesting that the increase in serum corticosterone concentration is associated with behavioral abnormality in zinc deficiency.

It is possible that HPA axis activity in zinc deficiency alter hippocampal function. The increase in serum corticosterone concentration increases corticosterone concentration in the brain extracellular fluid [103], followed by the increase in cytosolic free calcium concentration in neurons [84] (Figure 7).

In hippocampal slices from rats fed the zinc-deficient diet for 2 weeks, fura-2 signal was more than in the control hippocampal slices [102]. These results suggest that basal Ca^{2+} concentration in hippocampal cells is increased in association with the increase in serum corticosterone concentration. Glucocorticoids increase cytosolic Ca^{2+} concentration in cultured hippocampal neurons [104,105] and potentiate extracellular glutamate accumulation in the hippocampus [106,107]. Therefore, zinc-deficient mice and rats is a potential model to study pathological processes of psychological diseases.

REFERENCES

[1] Vallee, BL; Falchuk, KH. Zinc and gene expression. *Philos. Trans R. Soc. Lond B Biol. Sci.*, 1981, 294, 185-197.

[2] Coleman, JE. Zinc proteins: enzymes, storage proteins, transcription factors, and replication proteins. *Annu. Rev. Biochem*, 1992, 61, 897-946.

[3] Vallee, BL; Falchuk, KH. The biological basis of zinc physiology. *Physiol. Rev.*, 1993, 73, 79-118.

[4] Takeda, A. Movement of zinc and its functional significance in the brain. *Brain Res, Rev.*, 2000, 34, 137-148.

[5] Takeda, A. Essenttial trace metals and brain function. *Yakugaki Zasshi*, 2004, 124, 577-585.

[6] Haug, FMS. Heavy metals in the brain. A light microscope study of the rat with Timms' sulphide silver method. Methodological considerations and cytological and regional staining patterns. *Adv. Anat. Embryol. Cell Biol.*, 1973, 47, 1-71.

[7] Frederickson, CJ. Neurobiology of zinc and zinc-containing neurons. *Int. Rev. Neurobiol*, 1989, 31, 145-238.
[8] Takeda, A; Akiyama, T; Sawashita, J; Okada S: Brain uptake of trace metals, zinc and manganese, in rats. *Brain Res.*, 1994, 640, 341-344.
[9] Takeda, A. Zinc homeostasis and functions of zinc in the brain. *BioMetals*, 2001, 14, 343-352.
[10] Frederickson, CJ; Koh, JY; Bush, AI. The neurobiology of zinc in health and disease. *Nat. Rev. Neurosci*, 2005, 6, 449-462.
[11] Frederickson, CJ; Klitenick, MA; Manton, WI; Kirkpatrick, JB. Cytoarchitectonic distribution of zinc in the hippocampus of man and rat. *Brain Res.*, 1983, 273, 335-339.
[12] Sindreu, CB; Varoqui, H; Erickson, JD; Perez-Clausell, J. Boutons containing vesicular zinc define a subpopulation of synapses with low AMPAR content in rat hippocampus. *Cerebral Cortex*, 2003, 13, 823-829.
[13] Harrison, NL; Gibbons, SJ. Zn^{2+}: an endogenous modulator of ligend- and voltage-gated ion channels. *Neuropharmacolgy*, 1994, 33, 935-952.
[14] Smart, TG; Xie, X; Krishek, BJ. Modulation of inhibitory and excitatory amino acid receptor ion channels by zinc. *Prog. Neurobiol*, 1994, 42, 393-441.
[15] Huang, EP. Metal ions and synaptic transmission: think zinc. *Proc. Natl. Acad. Sci.*, 1997, 94, 13386-13387.
[16] Vogt, K; Mellor, J; Tong, G; Nicoll, R. The actions of synaptically released zinc at hippocampal mossy fiber synapses. *Neuron*, 2000, 26, 197-196.
[17] Li, Y; Hough, CJ; Suh, SW; Sarvey, JM; Frederickson, CJ. Rapid translocation of Zn(2+) from presynaptic terminals into postsynaptic hippocampal neurons after physiological stimulation. *J. Neurophysiol*, 2001, 86, 2597-2604.
[18] Assaf, SY; Chung, SH. Release of endogeneous Zn^{2+} from brain tissue during activity. *Nature*, 1984, 308, 734-735.
[19] Koh, JY; Suh, SW; Gwag, BJ; He, YY; Hsu, CY; Choi, DW. The role of zinc in selective neuronal death after transient global cerebral ischemia. *Science*, 1996, 272, 1013-1016.
[20] Choi, DW; Koh, JY. Zinc and brain injury. *Annu. Rev. Neurosci*, 1998, 21, 347-375.
[21] Lee, JM; Zipfel, GJ; Choi, DW. The changing landscape of ischaemic brain injury mechanisms. *Nature*, 1999, 399, A7-A14.

[22] Weiss, JH; Sensi, SL; Koh, JY. Zn(2+): a novel ionic mediator of neural injury in brain disease. *Trends Pharmacol. Sci.*, 2000, 21, 395-401.
[23] Suh, SW; Garnier, P; Aoyama, K; Chen, Y; Swanson, RA. Zinc release contributes to hypoglycemia-induced neuronal death. *Neurobiol. Dis.*, 2004, 16, 538-545.
[24] Takeda, A; Kawai, M; Okada, S. Zinc distribution in the brain of Nagase analbuminemic rat and enlargement of the ventricular system. *Brain Res.*, 1997, 769, 193-195.
[25] Aiken, SP; Horn, NR; Saunders, NR. Effect of histidine on tissue zinc distribution in rats. *BioMetals*, 1992, 5, 235-243.
[26] Takeda, A; Suzuki, M; Okada, S; Oku, N. Influence of histidine on zinc transport into rat brain. *J. Health Sci.*, 2000, 46, 209-213.
[27] Takeda, A; Suzuki, M; Oku, N. Possible involvement of plasma histidine in differential brain permeability to zinc and cadmium. *BioMetals*, 2002, 15, 371-375.
[28] Yamashita, T; Shimada, S; Guo, W; Sato, K; Kohmura, E; Hayakawa, T; Takagi, T; Tohyama, M. Cloning and functional expression of a brain peptide/histidene transporter. *J. Biol. Chem.*, 1997, 272, 10205-10211.
[29] Gunshin, H; Mackenzie, B; Berger, UV; Gunshin, Y; Romero, MF; Boron, WF; Nussberger, S; Gollan, JL; Hediger, MA. Cloning and characterization of a mammalian protein-coupled metal-ion transporter. *Nature*, 1997, 388, 482-488.
[30] Gaither, LA; Eide, DJ. Functional expression of the human hZIP2 zinc transporter. *J. Biol. Chem.*, 2000, 275, 5560-5564.
[31] Takeda, A; Sawashita, J; Okada, S. Biological half-lives of zinc and manganese in rat brain. *Brain Res.*, 1995, 695, 53-58.
[32] Takeda, A; Sawashita, J; Okada, S. Localization of rat brain of the trace metals, zinc and manganese, after intracerebroventricular injection. *Brain Res.*, 1994, 658, 252-254.
[33] Takeda, A; Suzuki, M; Okada, S; Oku, N. ^{65}Zn localization in rat brain after intracerebroventricular injection of ^{65}Zn-histidine. *Brain Res.*, 2000, 863, 241-244.
[34] Wensink, J; Molenaar, AJ; Woroniecka, UD; Van den Hamer, CJA. Zinc uptake into synaptosomes. *J. Neurochem*, 1988, 50, 782-789.
[35] Takeda, A; Fuke, S; Minami, A; Oku, N. Role of zinc influx via AMPA/kainate receptor activation in metabotropic glutamate receptor-mediated calcium release. *J. Neurosci. Res.*, 2007, 85, 1310-1317.

[36] Takeda, A; Fuke, S; Tsutsumi, W; Oku, N. Negative modulation of presynaptic activity by zinc released from Schaffer collaterals. *J. Neurosci. Res.*, in press.
[37] Takeda, A; Ohnuma, M; Sawashita, J; Okada, S. Zinc transport in the rat olfactory system. *Neurosci. Lett*, 1997, 225, 69-71.
[38] Takeda, A; Kodama, Y; Ohhuma, M; Okada, S. Zinc transport from the striatum and substantia nigra. *Brain Res. Bull.*, 1998, 47, 103-106.
[39] Takeda, A; Minami, A; Seki, Y; Oku, N. Differential Effects of Zinc on Glutamatergic and GABAergic Neurotransmitter Systems in the Hippocampus. *J. Neurosci. Res.*, 2004, 75, 225-229.
[40] Takeda, A; Minami, A; Seki, Y; Oku, N. Inhibitory function of zinc against excitation of hippocampal glutamatergic neurons. *Epilepsy Res.*, 2003, 57, 169-174.
[41] Rassendren, FA; Lory, P; Pin, JP; Nargeot, J. Zinc has opposite effects on NMDA and non-NMDA receptors expressed in Xenopus Oocytes. *Neuron*, 1990, 4, 733-740.
[42] Frederickson, CJ; Giblin, LJ; Krezel, A; McAdoo, DJ; Muelle, RN; Zeng, Y; Balaji, RV; Masalha, R; Thompson, RB; Fierke, CA; Sarvey, JM; Valdenebro, M; Prough, DS; Zornow, MH. Concentrations of extracellular free zinc (pZn)e in the central nervous system during simple anesthetization, ischemia and reperfusion. *Exp. Neurol*, 2006, 198, 285-293.
[43] Hirano, T; Kikuchi, K; Urano, Y; Higuchi, T; Nagano, T. Highly zinc-selective fluorescenct sensor molecules suitable for biological applications. *J. Am. Chem. Soc.*, 2000, 122, 12399-12400.
[44] Hirano, T; Kikuchi, K; Urano, Y; Nagano, T. Improvement and biological applications of fluorescent probes for zinc, ZnAFs. *J. Am. Chem. Soc.*, 2002, 124, 6555-6562.
[45] Minami, A; Sakurada, N; Fuke, S; Kikuchi, K; Nagano, T; Oku, N; Takeda, A. Inhibition of presynaptic activity by zinc released from mossy fiber terminals during tetanic stimulation. *J. Neurosci. Res.*, 2006, 83, 167-176.
[46] Lu, YM; Taverna, FA; Tu, R; Ackerley, CA; Wang, YT; Roder, J. Endogenous Zn(2+) is required for the induction of long-term potentiation at rat hippocampal mossy fiber-CA3 synapses. *Synapse*, 2000, 38, 187-197.
[47] Li, Y; Hough, CJ; Frederickson, CJ; Sarvey, JM. Induction of mossy fiber→CA3 long-term potentiation reguires translocation of synaptically released Zn2+. *J. Neurosci*, 2001, 21, 8015-8025.

[48] Cole, TB; Wenzel, HJ; Kafer, KE; Schwartzkroin, PA; Palmiter, RD. Elimination of zinc from synaptic vesicles in the intact mouse brain by disruption of the ZnT-3 gene. *Proc. Natl. Acad. Sci. USA*, 1999, 96, 1716-1721.
[49] Cole, TB; Robbins, CA; Wenzel, HJ; Schwartzkroin, PA; Palmiter, RD. Seizures and neuronal damage in mice lacking vesicular zinc. *Epilepsy Res.*, 2000, 39, 153-169.
[50] Xie, X; Smart, TG. Modulation of long-term potentiation in rat hippocampal pyramidal neurons by zinc. *Pflugers Arch.*, 1994, 427, 481-486.
[51] Klingauf, J; Kavalali, ET; Tsien, RW. Kinetics and regulation of fast endocytosis at hippocampal synapses. *Nature*, 1998, 394, 581-585.
[52] Zakharenko, SS; Zablow, L; Siegelbaum, SA. Visualization of changes in presynaptic function during long-term synaptic plasticity. *Nat. Neurosci*, 2001, 4, 711-717.
[53] Castillo, PE; Weisskopf, MG; Nicoll, RA. The role of Ca^{2+} channels in hippocampal mossy fiber synaptic transmission and long-term potentiation. *Neuron*, 1994, 12, 261-269.
[54] Nicoll, RA; Malenka, RC. Contrasting properties of two forms of long-term potentiation in the hippocampus. *Nature*, 1995, 377, 115-118.
[55] Breustedt, J; Vogt, KE; Miller, RJ; Nicoll, RA; Schmitz, D. Alpha1E-containing Ca^{2+} channels are involved in synaptic plasticity. *Proc. Natl. Acad. Sci. USA*, 2003, 100, 12450-12455.
[56] Wang, H; Storm, DR. Calmodulin-regulated adenylyl cyclases: cross-talk and plasticity in the central nervous system. *Mol. Pharmacol*, 2003, 63, 463-468.
[57] Takeda, A. Inhibitory modulatuon of glutamatergic neuron activity by zinc in the hippocampus. *Biomed. Res. Trace Elements*, 2006, 17, 399-405.
[58] Bancila, V; Nikonenko, I; Dunant, Y; Bloc, A. Zinc inhibits glutamate release via activation of pre-synaptic K_{ATP} channels and reduces ischaemic damage in rat hippocampus. *J. Neurochem*, 2004, 90, 1243-1250.
[59] Klein, C; Sunahara, RK; Hudson, TY; Heyduk, T; Howlett, AC. Zinc inhibition of camp signaling. *J. Biol. Chem.*, 2002, 277, 11859-11865.
[60] Kapur, A; Yeckel, MF; Johnston, D. L-type calcium channels are required for one form of hippocampal mossy fiber LTP. *J. Neurophysiol*, 1998, 79, 2181-2190.

[61] Bordi, F; Ugolini, A. Group I metabotropic glutamate receptors: implications for brain diseases. *Prog. Neurobiol*, 1999, 59, 55-79.
[62] Nicoletti, F; Bruno, V; Catania, MV; Battaglia, G; Copani, A; Barbagallo, G; Cena, V; Sanchez-Prieto, J; Spano, PF; Pizzi, M. Group-I metabotropic glutamate receptors: hypotheses to explain their dual role in neurotoxicity and neuroprotection. *Neuropharmacol*, 1999, 38, 1477-1484.
Favaron, M; Manev, RM; Candeo, P; Arban, R; Gabellini, N; Kozikowski, AP; Manev, H. Trans-azetidine-2,4-dicarboxylic acid activates neuronal metabotropic receptors. *NeuroReport*, 1993, 4, 967-970.
[63] Riedel, G; Manahan-Vaughan, D; Kozikowski, AP; Reymann, KG. Metabotropic glutamate receptor agonist trans-azetidine-2,4-dicarboxylic acid facilitates maintenance of LTP in the dentate gyrus in vivo. *Neuropharmacol*, 1995, 34, 1107-1109.
[64] Riedel, G; Wetzel, W; Reymann, KG. Metabotropic glutamate receptors in spatial and nonspatial learning in rats studied by means of agonist and antagonist application. *Learn Mem.*, 1995, 2, 243-265.
[65] Sensi, SL; Canzoniero, LMT; Yu, SP; Ying, HS; Koh, JY; Kerchner, GA; Choi, DW. Measurement of intracellular free zinc in living cortical neurons: routes of entry. *J. Neurosci*, 1997, 15, 9554-9564.
[66] Schmidt-Kastner, R; Freund, TF. Selective vulnerability of the hippocampus in brain ischemia. *Neuroscience*, 1991, 40, 599-636.
[67] Liu, S; Lau, L; Wei, J; Zhu, D; Zou, S; Sun, H; Fu, Y; Liu, F; Lu, Y. Expression of Ca2+-permeable AMPA receptor channels primes cell death in transient forebrain ischemia. *Neuron*, 2004, 43, 43-55.
[68] Takeda, A; Minami, A; Sakurada, N; Nakajima, S; Oku, N. Response of hippocampal mossy fiber zinc to excessive glutamate release. *Neurochem. Int.*, 2007, 50, 322-327.
[69] Rodriguez-Moreno, A; Sihra, TS. Presynaptic kainate receptor facilitation of glutamate release involves protein kinase A in the rat hippocampus. *J. Physiol.*, 2004, 557, 733-745.
[70] Levi, G; Patrizio, M. Astrocytes heterogeneity: endogenous amino acid levels and release evoked by non-N-methyl-D-aspartate receptor agonists and by potassium-induced swelling in type-1 and type-2 astrocytes. *J. Neurochem*, 1992, 58, 1943-1952.
[71] Takeda, A; Nakajima, S; Fuke, S; Sakurada, N; Minami, A; Oku, N. Zinc release from Schaffer collaterals and its significance. *Brain Res. Bull.*, 2006, 68, 442-447.

[72] Takeda, A; Hirate, M; Tamano, H; Oku, N. Zinc movement in the brain under kainate-induced seizures. *Epilepsy Res.*, 2003, 54, 123-129.
[73] Sloviter, R. A selective loss of hippocampal mossy fiber Timm stain accompanies granule cell seizure activity induced by perforant path stimulation. *Brain Res.*, 1985, 330, 150-153.
[74] Frederickson, CJ; Hernandez, MD; Goik, SA; Morton, JD; McGinty, JF: Loss of zinc staining from hippocampal mossy fibers during kainic acid induced seizures: a histofluorescence study. *Brain Res.*, 1988, 446, 383-386.
[75] Takeda, A; Hirate, M; Tamano, H; Nishibaba, D; Oku, N. Susceptibility to kainate-induced seizures under dietary zinc deficiency. *J. Neurochem*, 2003, 85, 1575-1580.
[76] Takeda, A; Tamano, H; Nagayoshi, A; Yamada, K; Oku, N. Increase in hippocampal cell death after treatment with kainate in zinc deficiency. *Neurochem. Int.*, 2005, 47, 539-544.
[77] Biondi, M; Picardi, A. Psychological stress and neuroendocrine function in humans: the last two decades of research. *Psychother Psychosom*, 1999, 68, 114-150.
[78] Negrao, AB; Deuster, PA; Gold, PW; Singh, A; Chrousos, GP. Individual reactivity and physiology of the stress response. *Biomed. Pharmacother*, 2000, 54, 122-128.
[79] Hennessy, MB; Levine, S. Sensitive pituitary-adrenal responsiveness to varying intensities of psychological stimulation. *Physiol. Behav*, 1978, 21, 295-297.
[80] Armario, A; Lopez-Calderon, A; Jolin, T; Castellanos, JM. Sensitivity of anterior pituitary hormones to graded levels of psychological stress. *Life Sci.*, 1986, 39, 471-475.
[81] Dai, H; Krost, M; Carey, RJ. A new methodological approach to the study of habituation: the use of positive and negative behavioral indices of habituation. *J. Neurosci. Methods*, 1995, 62, 169-174.
[82] Whishaw, IQ; Vanderwolf, CH. Hippocampal EEG and behavior: changes in amplitude and frequency of RSA (theta rhythm) associated with spontaneous and learned movement patternsin rats and cats. *Behav. Biol.*, 1973, 8, 461-484.
[83] Lee, AL; Ogle, WO; Sapolsky, RM. Stress and depression: possible links to neuron death in the hippocampus. *Bipolar Disorders*, 2002, 4, 117-128.

[84] Takeda, A; Sakurada, N; Kanno, S; Minami, A; Oku, N. Response of extracelluar zinc in the ventral hippocampus against novelty stress. *J. Neurochem*, 2006, 99, 670-676.
[85] Brown, KH; Wuehler, SE; Peerson, JM. The importance of zinc in human nutrition and estimation of the global prevalence of zinc deficiency. *Food Nutri. Bull*, 2001, 22, 113-125.
[86] Golub, MS; Keen, CL; Gershwin, ME; Hendrickx, AG. Developmental zinc deficiency and behavior. *J. Nutr.*, 1995, 125, 2263-2271.
[87] Sandstead, HH; Frederickson, CJ; Penland, JG. History of zinc as related to brain function. *J. Nutr.*, 2000, 130, 496S-502S.
[88] Prohaska, JR; Luecke, RW; Jasinski, R. Effect of zinc deficiency from day 18 of gestation and/or during lactation on the development of some rat brain enzymes. *J. Nutr.*, 1974, 104, 1525-1531.
[89] Takeda, A; Hirate, M; Tamano, H; Oku, N. Release of glutamate and GABA in the hippocampus under zinc deficiency. *J. Neurosci. Res.*, 2003, 72, 537-542.
[90] Takeda, A; Minami, A; Takefuta, S; Tochigi, M; Oku, N. Zinc homeostasis in the brain of adult rats fed zinc-deficient diet. *J. Neurosci. Res.*, 2001, 63, 447-452.
[91] Sterman, MB; Shouse, MN; Fairchild, MD. Zinc and seizure mechanisms. In Morley, J.E., Sterman M.B., and Walsh J.H., (Eds.), *Nutritional modulation of neural function*, Academic Press, San Diego, 1988, 307-319.
[92] Takeda, A; Hanajima, T; Ijiro, H; Ishige, A; Iizuka, S; Okada, S; Oku, N. Release of zinc from the brain of El (epilepsy) mice during seizure induction. *Brain Res.*, 1999, 828, 174-178.
[93] Hirate, M; Takeda, A; Tamano, H; Enomoto, S; Oku, N. Distribution of trace elements in the brain of EL (epilepsy) mice. *Epilepsy Res.*, 2002, 51, 109-116.
[94] Takeda, A; Hirate, M; Oku, N. Elimination of zinc-65 from the brain under kainate-induced seizures. *BioMetals*, 2004, 17, 141-144.
[95] Takeda, A; Tamano, H; Oku, N. Involvement of Unusual Glutamate Release in kainate-induced seizures in zinc-deficient adult rats. *Epilepsy Res.*, 2005, 66, 137-143.
[96] Lipton, SA; Rosenberg, PA. Excitatory amino acids as a final common pathway for neurologic disorders. *N. Engl. J. Med.*, 1994, 330, 613-622.
[97] Obrenovitch, TP; Urenjak, J. Altered glutamatergic transmission in neurological disorders: from high extracellular glutamate to excessive synaptic efficacy. *Prog. Neurobiol*, 1997, 51, 39-87.

[98] Reeves, PG; Frissell, SG; O'Dell, BL. Response of serum corticosterone to ACTH and stress in the zinc-deficient rat. *Proc. Soc. Exp. Biol. Med*, 1997, 156, 500-504.

[99] Gaetke, LM; Frederick, RC; Oz, HS; McClain, CJ. Decreased food intake rather than zinc deficiency is associated with changes in plasma leptin, metabolic rate, and activity levels in zinc deficient rats. *J. Nutr. Biochem*, 2002, 13, 237-244.

[100] Chu, Y; Mouat, MF; Harris, RBS; Coffield, JA; Grider, A. Water maze performance and changes in serum corticosterone levels in zinc-deprived and pair-fed rats. *Physiol. Behav.*, 2003, 78, 569-578.

[101] Takeda, A; Tamano, H; Kan, F; Itoh, H; Oku, N. Anxiety-like Behavior of Young Rats after 2-Week Zinc Deprivation. *Behav. Brain Res.*, 2007, 177, 1-6.

[102] Cook, CJ. Glucocorticoid feedback increases the sensitivity of the limbic system to stress. *Physiol. Behav*, 2002, 75, 455-464.

[103] Elliott, EM; Sapolsky, RM. Corticosterone enhances kainic acid-induced calcium elevation in cultured hippocampal neurons. *J. Neurochem*, 1992, 59, 1033-1040.

[104] Elliott, EM; Sapolsky, RM. Corticosterone impairs hippocampal neuronal calcium regulation – possible mediating mechanisms. *Brain Res.*, 1993, 602, 84-90.

[105] Stein-Behrens, BA; Elliott, EM; Miller, CA; Schilling, JW; Newcombe, R; Sapolsky, RM. Glucocorticoids exacerbate kainic acid-induced extracellular accumulation of excitatory amino acids in the rat hippocampus. *J. Neurochem*, 1992, 58, 1730-1735.

[106] Stein-Behrens, BA; Lin, WJ; Sapolsky, RM. Physiological elevation of glucocorticoids potentiates glutamate accumulation in the hippocampus. *J. Neurochem*, 1994, 63, 596-602.

INDEX

A

Abraham, 116
abuse, 49, 50, 62, 64, 69, 72, 73, 130, 131, 132, 137, 138, 140, 141, 145
AC, 171
accidents, 126
acetylcholine, 109, 111, 122
acid, viii, 2, 11, 18, 20, 27, 28, 29, 31, 33, 35, 43, 65, 70, 107, 120, 127, 145, 150, 168, 172, 173, 175
ACTH, 175
action potential, 2, 47, 80, 127, 130, 135, 159
activation, 127, 129, 139, 142, 146, 159, 160, 162, 163, 165, 167, 169, 171
activity level, vii, 2, 19, 22, 114, 175
acute stress, 134
AD, 23, 24, 71, 104, 105, 106, 123
adaptation, 31, 40, 69, 131, 139, 145
adaptations, 52, 72, 138, 139, 141
addiction, ix, x, 125, 126, 127, 132, 133, 137, 139, 142, 145, 146, 147
adenylyl cyclase, 171
adhesion, 16, 30, 115
adjustment, vii, 2
administration, 130, 131, 132, 133, 135, 136, 137, 138, 139, 141, 142, 143, 144, 145, 147

adrenoceptors, 105, 119
adult, 174
AE, 142
age, 47, 105, 106, 112
aggregation, 25, 37
agonist, 9, 86, 136, 164, 172
AJ, 143, 169
akinesia, 25
AL, 173
Albert Einstein, 125
albumin, 151, 152
alcohol dependence, 71
algorithm, 69
alpha, 127
ALS, 10, 17
alters, 67, 70, 71, 140, 142, 143, 146, 147
Alzheimer's disease, x, 149, 166
AM, 140, 142, 143, 144
amino, viii, 8, 22, 28, 36, 43, 65, 70, 84, 107, 127, 145, 147, 150, 151, 152, 156, 168, 172, 174, 175
amino acid, 8, 22, 84, 145, 147, 151, 152, 156, 168, 172, 174, 175
amino acids, 8, 22, 147, 151, 152, 156, 174, 175
AMPA, 127, 128, 129, 130, 131, 132, 133, 135, 136, 140, 143, 144, 145, 146, 147, 150, 155, 160, 161, 162, 169, 172

AMPAR potentiation, viii, 43, 45, 54, 58, 60, 62, 63
amplitude, 2, 12, 15, 19, 22, 38, 40, 45, 47, 58, 59, 63, 81, 135, 173
amygdala, 34, 35, 61, 71, 126, 128, 152, 154
amyloid beta, 23, 33, 34, 119
amyotrophic lateral sclerosis, x, 10, 17, 149, 166
anatomy, 131
anesthetization, 170
animal models, 139, 145
animals, 128, 130, 131, 133, 135, 136, 137, 138, 139, 150, 151, 165
anorexia, 166
ANOVA, 50
antagonist, 131, 132, 133, 134, 143, 160, 172
antagonists, 132, 136, 137
anterior pituitary, 173
antibody, 55
antipsychotic, 85
antisense, 91
anxiety, viii, 27, 36, 43, 44, 46, 54, 57, 58, 60, 61, 62, 63, 65, 68, 164, 167
Anxiety, 175
AP, 172
apoptosis, 25, 39, 103
AR, 145
arginine, 10, 17
arousal, 65, 164
AS, 142
aspartate, viii, 44, 65, 70, 71, 72, 117, 120, 127, 142, 150, 172
aspartic acid, 81
astrocytes, 26, 172
ATP, 159
atrophy, 90
attention, 126, 164
attribution, 134
auditory cortex, 104, 117
autism, ix, 23, 76, 79, 80, 85, 92, 97
autosomal dominant, 25
autosomal recessive, 25, 33
availability, 137

aversion, 138, 142
axon terminals, ix, 75, 77, 80, 82, 91
axonal, 154
axons, 89

B

barbiturates, viii, 44, 49, 52, 61, 62, 72
barrier, 150, 151, 152
barriers, 152
basal ganglia, 104, 109, 118, 120
base, 89
behavior, 133, 138, 139, 142, 144, 145, 146, 158, 164, 165, 167, 173, 174
behavioral change, 146
behavioral modification, 138
behavioral sensitization, 72, 133, 134, 137, 140, 143, 146, 147
behaviors, 44, 64, 83, 125, 130, 132, 133, 134, 135, 137, 139
beneficial effect, 115
benzodiazepine, viii, 43, 44, 45, 49, 54, 55, 61, 62, 63, 64, 65, 66, 69, 70, 71, 73
benzodiazepine anxiolytics, viii, 43
bias, 117
bicarbonate, 63, 69
binding, 127, 128, 151, 156
bipolar disorder, ix, 76, 84, 98
blocks, 132, 133, 144
blood, 24, 152
blood-brain barrier, 152
body temperature, vii, 1
Boron, 169
boutons, 150, 157, 159
brain functions, 23
brain injury, 168
brainstem, 105, 118
branching, 81
brevis, 114
Butcher, 96
butyric, 150

Index

C

Ca^{2+} signals, 76, 79
cadmium, 156, 169
calcium channels, x, 149, 153, 156, 159, 160, 171
calmodulin, 127, 159
cAMP, 159
cancer, 93
candidates, 102, 104, 152
cannabinoids, 145
capillary, 152
car accidents, 126
carbamazepine, 132
carrier, 153
cascades, 6, 11, 12, 57, 128
casein, 55
caspases, 103
cation, 54
cats, 173
CB, 168
CD, 145
cell, 127, 128, 130, 147, 150, 155, 156, 157, 158, 160, 161, 162, 163, 164, 166, 172, 173
cell biology, vii, 94, 96
cell culture, 12
cell death, 12, 24, 25, 29, 79, 172, 173
cell division, 150
cell surface, 18
central nervous system, 8, 93, 116, 170, 171
cerebellar development, 97
cerebellum, 153
cerebral cortex, 72, 140
cerebral ischemia, 168
cerebrospinal fluid, 150
challenges, 10, 17
channel blocker, 2, 154
channels, x, 129, 131, 132, 135, 149, 153, 156, 159, 160, 168, 171, 172
chemical, 9, 107
chemokines, 26
China, 29
chorea, 120
choroid, 151, 152
CK, 142, 144
CL, 174
classes, 47, 62
classroom, 126
cleavage, 23
clinical assessment, 119
clusters, 3
CNQX, 160
CNS, viii, 17, 44, 49, 52, 62, 71, 97, 115
cocaine, 21, 49, 64, 68, 72, 130, 131, 132, 133, 134, 135, 136, 137, 138, 139, 140, 141, 142, 143, 144, 145, 146, 147
codon, 10, 17
cognitive, 133, 158, 165
cognitive deficit, 121
cognitive deficits, 121
cognitive function, 16, 93, 133
cognitive impairment, 105, 106
cognitive performance, 115, 123
cognitive process, 165
collateral, 45, 89, 90, 150, 163
color, iv, 77
communication, 102, 104
compensation, 35
competition, 21
complexity, 94
components, 135
composition, 10, 17, 21, 22, 29, 30, 39, 70
compounds, 62, 69
compulsion, 142
concentration, 150, 151, 153, 154, 156, 159, 161, 164, 165, 166, 167
conditioning, 34, 114, 134
conductance, 45, 47, 63, 69
conduction, 127
Congress, iv, 121
connectivity, 2, 79, 116
consolidation, 15, 116
consumption, 109
control, 132, 136, 146, 166, 167
control group, 166
convergence, 107
copyright, iv
Copyright, iv
correlation, 47, 111, 113

cortex, 12, 14, 19, 30, 33, 39, 47, 82, 86, 89, 104, 105, 107, 108, 109, 110, 111, 112, 114, 117, 118, 120, 121, 122, 123, 126, 138, 140, 141, 142, 143, 144, 145, 146, 147, 153, 154, 155
cortical, 128
cortical neurons, 5, 14, 21, 32, 49, 61, 68, 71, 72, 87, 88, 89, 92, 172
corticosterone, 166, 167, 175
Corticosterone, 175
CPP, 132, 133, 134
CR, 147
craving, 126, 133
crosstalk, x, 149, 150, 151
cross-talk, 171
CSF, 152, 153
CST, 89, 90
C-terminus, 128
cues, 126, 133, 134
culture, 12, 19, 87
culture medium, 87
cycling, 141
cysteine, 151, 152
cytokines, 26, 115
cytomegalovirus, 89
cytoplasm, 78, 86
cytosolic, 156, 167
cytotoxicity, 87, 88

D

damages, iv
death, 168, 169, 172, 173
deaths, 105
decay, 50, 52, 58, 105
declarative memory, 105
deep brain stimulation, 115
deficiencies, 25
deficiency, ix, x, 101, 105, 150, 151, 165, 166, 167, 173, 174, 175
deficit, 28
degenerate, 77, 162
degradation, 6, 7, 11, 12, 22, 24, 29, 30, 31, 32, 33, 53, 88, 140
delivery, 127, 146, 158, 161, 162, 163

delta, 144
dementia, 25, 105, 121
dendrites, ix, 3, 4, 7, 19, 22, 28, 47, 75, 76, 78, 79, 82, 89, 91, 94, 95
dendritic spines, 28, 71, 76, 77, 78, 79, 81, 82, 86, 94, 95, 111, 123
density, 143, 144, 146
dentate gyrus, 152, 161, 172
dephosphorylation, 33
depolarization, 6, 47, 50, 54, 63, 68, 112, 127, 144, 154, 158, 159, 160
deposits, 108
depressants, viii, 44, 49, 52, 62
depressed, 136
depression, 3, 14, 24, 25, 28, 31, 33, 34, 36, 38, 55, 58, 80, 95, 113, 117, 119, 127, 129, 136, 141, 142, 143, 145, 146, 162, 173
deprivation, 5, 6, 11, 12, 14, 17, 18, 19, 165, 167
depth, 115
derivatives, 84
desensitization, 80, 93
desynchronization, 106
detection, 121
diamonds, 51
diet, 165, 167, 174
dietary, 165, 173
differentiation, 150
diffusion, 34, 54, 79
disability, 111
discharges, 164
disease model, 67
diseases, 24, 106, 114, 119, 166, 167, 172
disorder, ix, 24, 77, 85, 102, 106, 109, 110, 111, 174
displacement, 55
distress, 109
distribution, 32, 56, 67, 93, 151, 168, 169
diversity, 64
division, 150
dominance, 12, 39
dopamine, ix, 64, 68, 72, 76, 77, 79, 80, 83, 85, 92, 93, 97, 99, 109, 111, 116, 119,

Index

121, 128, 140, 141, 142, 144, 145, 146, 147
dopaminergic, 21, 104, 105, 106, 107, 108, 109, 110, 126, 130, 140, 143, 145, 146
dopaminergic neurons, 130, 145
dorsolateral prefrontal cortex, 84
down-regulation, viii, 3, 14, 20, 22, 24, 26, 44, 84
Drosophila, 78
drug abuse, 64
drug addict, 23, 126, 139
drug addiction, 23, 126, 139
drug exposure, 126, 130, 135, 137, 139
drug targets, 62, 92
drug treatment, 2, 49, 52
drug use, ix, x, 125, 126
drug withdrawal, 45, 46, 49, 55, 61, 62
drug-induced, ix, x, 125, 127, 130, 131, 133, 136, 137, 138, 139
drug-related, 125, 133, 134
drugs, 49, 50, 52, 62, 69, 72, 97, 126, 128, 130, 131, 132, 133, 137, 138, 140, 144
duration, 131
dyes, 86
dystonia, ix, 101, 102, 110, 111, 112, 114, 115, 122

E

early postnatal development, 10
editors, 121
EEG, 106, 119, 173
Einstein, 125
electrodes, 131
electron, 45, 56, 57, 67, 70
electrophysiological, 130, 135, 140
elongation, 22, 93
EM, 140, 142, 144, 175
e-mail, 101
EMG, 90
emotion, ix, x, 125, 126, 139
emotional, 158
emotional memory, 126
emotional state, 126, 139
emotions, 126

encoding, 88
endocytosis, 171
endogenous, 136
endothelial cell, 152
endothelial cells, 152
enlargement, 169
entorhinal cortex, 153, 154
environment, vii, 1, 12, 83, 142, 164
environmental, 133, 140
environmental context, 133, 140
environmental stress, 87
environments, 83, 116
enzymes, 77, 79, 86, 150, 167, 174
epilepsy, x, 14, 149, 164, 166, 174
epileptic seizures, 164, 165
episodic memory, 158
epithelial cell, 151
epithelial cells, 151
equilibrium, 136
ER, 142
ET, 171
ethanol, viii, 44, 49, 51, 52, 61, 62, 68, 71, 72, 130, 132, 144
Ethanol, 132
etiology, 165
evidence, ix, x, 15, 19, 24, 25, 26, 46, 55, 61, 67, 70, 101, 103, 104, 107, 111, 112, 115, 122, 125, 126, 129, 130, 136, 137, 142, 150, 158
evoked potential, 110, 114, 117
excitability, 2, 26, 44, 70, 105, 111, 113, 115, 135, 138, 144
excitation, ix, 2, 6, 13, 23, 31, 54, 102, 111, 112, 115, 153, 156, 159, 160, 161, 162, 163, 164, 170
excitatory postsynaptic potentials, 86
excitatory synapses, ix, x, 15, 28, 32, 38, 40, 125, 126, 127, 129, 131, 135, 136, 138, 139, 140, 142
excitotoxicity, x, 23, 34, 112, 120, 149, 150, 151, 162, 166
execution, 23
executive function, 84, 109
executive functions, 84

exocytosis, 9, 16, 25, 34, 37, 81, 84, 97, 158, 159
exogenous, 136
explicit memory, 126
exposure, ix, x, 21, 49, 52, 54, 61, 68, 72, 125, 126, 130, 131, 132, 133, 135, 136, 137, 138, 139, 140, 141, 142, 143, 144, 146
Exposure, 126
extinction, 132
extracellular, 130, 135, 150, 154, 155, 156, 159, 160, 162, 164, 165, 166, 167, 170, 174, 175
extracellular matrix, 30

F

FA, 170
FAD, 27
families, 87
fascia, 95, 116
fat, 121
fat intake, 121
fatty acids, 109
fear, 34, 126, 145, 164
feedback, x, 129, 138, 149, 175
female rat, 144
femur, 165
fiber, 110, 156, 157, 158, 159, 160, 162, 168, 170, 171, 172, 173
fibers, 89, 90, 150, 154, 156, 157, 158, 159, 160, 162, 164, 173
fish, 87
fluid, 150, 154, 156, 167
fluorescence, 4, 156
fluoxetine, 132
food, 126, 166, 175
food intake, 175
force, 70
Ford, 72
forebrain, 37, 49, 172
formation, 15, 16, 18, 21, 23, 31, 70, 81, 84, 98, 125, 126, 127, 161
free radicals, 86
frequenin, 93, 95

frontal cortex, 49, 99, 106
functional analysis, 99
fusion, 9, 34

G

GABA, 39, 44, 51, 52, 54, 62, 63, 64, 69, 130, 144, 150, 154, 156, 163, 166, 174
GABAergic, 126, 128, 132, 140, 154, 170
ganglion, 91
GC, 142
GE, 147
gene, 167, 171
gene expression, 47, 71, 115, 167
genes, 109
genetics, 97
gestation, 174
GL, 141
glia, 11, 12, 26
glial, 153
glial cells, 12, 26, 153
glucocorticoid, 92, 105, 132, 144
glucocorticoid receptor, 132
glucocorticoids, 92, 105, 175
glutamatergic, 128, 133, 141, 145, 146, 150, 154, 158, 164, 165, 170, 171, 174
glutamine, 10, 17, 26, 87
glycine, 9
goal-directed, 139
goal-directed behavior, 139
goals, 127
granule cells, 154, 162
granules, 35
groups, 130
growth, 16, 30, 81, 84, 91, 93, 96, 102, 165, 166
growth factor, 84, 91
GTPases, 16, 30
guanine, 4
gyrus, 152, 161, 172

H

habituation, 173
health, 168

Health and Human Services, 64
heart, 126
heart rate, 126
heavy metal, 156
heavy metals, 156
heterogeneity, 115, 172
hippocampal, 126, 127, 128, 129, 131, 141, 146, 147, 150, 152, 153, 154, 155, 156, 158, 159, 162, 163, 164, 165, 167, 168, 170, 171, 172, 173, 175
hippocampus, vii, ix, x, 25, 33, 36, 37, 40, 44, 45, 47, 67, 83, 86, 98, 101, 102, 104, 107, 113, 116, 118, 128, 129, 149, 150, 152, 153, 154, 155, 164, 165, 166, 167, 168, 171, 172, 173, 174, 175
Hippocampus, 149, 170
histidine, 151, 152, 153, 169
history, 113, 114, 146
HIV, 89, 90
homeostasis, 4, 20, 25, 30, 31, 35, 94, 112, 115, 122, 164, 165, 168, 174
homeostatic mechanism, vii, 1, 4, 7, 114
Homeostatic regulation, vii, 1, 32, 34
hormones, 144, 173
House, 146
HPA, 164, 166, 167
HPA axis, 164, 166, 167
human, ix, 26, 30, 89, 101, 104, 111, 114, 116, 117, 118, 120, 123, 164, 169, 174
human brain, 104
human immunodeficiency virus, 89
humans, 165, 173
hybridization, 135, 153
hydration levels, vii, 1
hydrogen, 88
hydrogen peroxide, 88
hydrolysis, 161
hydrolyzed, 156
hydroxyl, 36
hyperactivity, 2, 24
hypoglycemia, 169
hypokinesia, 109
hypothalamus, 153
hypothesis, 102, 118

I

identification, 127
image, 155, 157
images, 56, 57
immune activation, 12
immune response, 12
immunohistochemistry, 80
impairments, 110
implicit memory, 105
impulsive, 138
in situ, 135
in situ hybridization, 54, 135
in vitro, 4, 15, 49, 61, 81, 85, 136, 145, 147
in vivo, 12, 15, 19, 28, 37, 38, 49, 52, 54, 61, 67, 76, 80, 81, 86, 97, 98, 105, 115, 119, 131, 132, 141, 146, 150, 154, 161, 172
indicators, 158
indices, 173
individual differences, 142
individuals, 37, 126
induction, ix, 7, 8, 11, 12, 18, 26, 31, 36, 83, 101, 103, 104, 112, 113, 131, 133, 136, 137, 146, 158, 159, 170, 174
ineffectiveness, 47
infancy, 165
inflammation, 12
ingestion, 71
inhibition, ix, 2, 7, 13, 22, 23, 47, 51, 52, 53, 65, 102, 106, 111, 115, 122, 140, 156, 159, 163, 171
inhibitor, 88, 89, 107, 132, 138, 146
inhibitory, 126, 128, 130, 158, 168
initiation, 12, 13, 19
injection, 152, 153, 169
injections, 90
injuries, vii, 1, 26, 105
injury, iv, 26, 77, 81, 84, 88, 90, 91, 94, 111, 118, 122, 168, 169
injury mechanisms, 168
inner ear, 99
inositol, 78
insertion, viii, 5, 6, 9, 10, 11, 15, 18, 34, 35, 36, 43, 54, 62, 63, 82, 96, 130

integration, 147
integrin, 11, 17, 18
integrins, 17, 29, 115
integrity, 23
interaction, 128
Interaction, 144
interactions, 144, 146
interference, 85
internalization, 5, 6, 7, 9, 10, 11, 18, 19, 21, 22, 34, 35, 54, 80, 128, 129, 130
interneuron, 10, 38
interneurons, 14, 35, 120, 156, 163
INTRACELLULAR CALCIUM, 13, 24, 156, 160, 162, 163
intracellular signaling, 127, 128
intravenous, 152
intrinsic, 138, 139, 141
ion channels, 33, 54, 78, 131, 168
ion transport, 169
ionic, 138, 169
ionotropic glutamate receptor, 160
ions, 127, 168
IQ, 173
iron, 32
ischemia, x, 10, 17, 31, 36, 37, 149, 162, 166, 168, 170, 172
ischemic, 161

J

Japan, 121, 149
JT, 141

K

K^+, 69
kainate receptor, 150, 155, 160, 161, 162, 169, 172
kainic acid, 173, 175
KH, 167, 174
kinase, 127, 129, 142, 172
kinases, 127
kinetics, 81

L

LA, 169
labeling, 56, 57, 79, 157
lactation, 174
landscape, 168
laser, 155, 157
lateral sclerosis, x, 149, 166
LC, 144
lead, viii, 6, 11, 23, 54, 75, 76, 79, 92, 111, 112, 113, 114, 126, 158
learning, viii, ix, x, 3, 4, 29, 40, 75, 76, 80, 81, 83, 86, 91, 95, 97, 99, 102, 103, 104, 107, 111, 112, 118, 125, 126, 134, 137, 138, 139, 142, 143, 144, 147, 158, 172
leptin, 175
lesions, 90, 120
LEUKOCYTES, 98
lice, 145
ligand, 13, 55, 61, 78, 151
ligands, 151, 156
light, 7, 22, 32, 39, 67, 115, 167
limbic system, 175
links, 173
liver, 165
LM, 143, 175
localization, 6, 11, 17, 31, 32, 55, 66, 67, 78, 79, 82, 89, 93, 169
locomotor, 133, 134, 164
locomotor activity, 134, 164
locus, 87
long period, 133
Long Term Depression, ix, 79, 101, 103, 111
Long Term Potentiation (LTP), vii, ix, 79, 101, 102
long- term synaptic plasticity, viii, 75, 76, 92
long-term, 127, 132, 141, 142, 143, 144, 145, 146
long-term potentiation, 127, 141, 143, 144, 146, 158, 170, 171
Long-term potentiation, 145
low molecular weight, 156
LSM, 155, 157

LTD, vii, ix, 3, 4, 8, 9, 10, 21, 27, 34, 36, 79, 80, 82, 85, 86, 96, 98, 101, 103, 105, 106, 107, 111, 112, 113, 114, 119, 127, 128, 129, 130, 131, 135, 136, 137, 143, 162
LTP, 127, 128, 129, 130, 131, 133, 134, 136, 138, 139, 143, 158, 159, 161, 171, 172
lysine, 8, 22

M

machinery, 9, 22, 29
magnesium, 103, 127, 156
magnetic resonance, 104
magnitude, 111, 112, 136
maintenance, 129, 132, 137, 161, 172
majority, 8, 106
mammalian brain, vii, 1, 76
mammals, 78
man, 168
management, 14, 122
manganese, 168, 169
MANOVA, 56, 57
MAPK, 143
matter, iv, 150
maturation, 165
MB, 142, 173, 174
measurement, 81, 130
medial prefrontal cortex, 141, 143, 144, 145, 146
median, 108, 110
mediation, 78, 91
membranes, 16, 49, 151
memory, viii, ix, x, 3, 4, 15, 17, 23, 36, 40, 52, 75, 76, 80, 81, 83, 85, 86, 91, 97, 98, 102, 105, 106, 107, 109, 112, 118, 120, 125, 126, 138, 139, 140, 158, 161
memory formation, 17, 83, 161
memory function, 106, 118, 158
mental retardation, ix, 20, 33, 36, 76, 84, 85, 91, 97
messenger RNA, 35
messengers, 94
metabolic, 175

metabolic rate, 175
metabolism, 25
metabotropic glutamate receptor, 160, 163, 169, 172
metabotropic glutamate receptors, 129, 135, 160, 163, 172
metalloproteins, 150, 165
metals, 156, 167, 168, 169
methodology, 111, 146
Mg^{2+}, 60
mice, 12, 16, 19, 20, 21, 23, 24, 26, 29, 30, 31, 33, 36, 70, 73, 79, 83, 85, 97, 99, 103, 107, 111, 117, 131, 134, 141, 142, 144, 145, 152, 158, 164, 165, 167, 171, 174
microdialysis, 150, 153, 154
microinjection, 136
microorganisms, 150
microscope, 167
midbrain, 72, 126, 131, 134, 140, 143, 145
miniature, 2, 45, 135
mitochondria, 87
mitogen, 66
MK-80, 142
models, ix, 26, 32, 37, 45, 62, 101, 107, 109, 112, 113, 114, 116, 119, 121, 122, 123, 127, 139, 145, 164
modifications, vii, 1, 4, 26, 50, 112, 117
modulation, 131, 137, 138, 142, 143, 144, 147, 154, 158, 159, 162, 163, 170, 174
molecular mechanisms, 127, 128, 136, 142
molecular weight, 156
molecules, 6, 13, 16, 17, 18, 26, 30, 86, 92, 115, 170
morphine, 49, 62, 68, 130, 132, 134, 145, 147
morphological, 147
morphology, 16, 37, 76, 79, 103
motivation, 104, 126, 139
motor behavior, 111
motor control, 118
motor task, 111
mouse, 171
movement, 164, 173
MR, 142

186 Index

mRNA, 8, 19, 20, 37, 39, 49, 54, 61, 72, 83, 135, 143, 151, 153
mRNAs, 26, 31, 38
MS, 174
muscle contraction, 110
musicians, 122
mutant, 16, 20, 22, 25, 26, 31, 85, 87, 92, 98, 122, 144
mutation, 85, 87, 151
mutations, 27, 38, 87, 99
MV, 172

N

N- methyl-D-aspartate receptors (NMDAR), viii
Na+, 127
naming, 109
National Academy of Sciences, 36, 93, 94
National Institutes of Health, 27
natural, 126, 128
NCS, viii, 75, 76, 77, 78, 79, 80, 81, 82, 83, 84, 85, 86, 87, 88, 89, 90, 91, 92, 93, 94, 96, 98, 99
necrosis, 12, 33, 36, 38
negative consequences, ix, x, 125, 126
negative feedback response, vii, 1
neocortex, 47
nerve, 25, 29, 88, 96, 105, 108, 110, 118, 121, 137
nervous system, vii, 1, 13, 14, 16, 20, 35, 37, 39, 170, 171
neural development, 112
neural function, 174
neural network, 6, 26
neural networks, 26
neural system, 112
neural systems, 112
neurobehavioral, 140
neurobiology, 94, 95, 96, 142, 145, 168
neuroblastoma, 159
neurodegeneration, vii, 27, 29, 87, 92, 94, 99, 113, 154, 160, 164
neurodegenerative, 160
neurodegenerative diseases, 22, 30

neurodegenerative disorders, ix, 76
neurodegenerative processes, 160
neuroendocrine, 173
neuroendocrine cells, 78
neurofibrillary tangles, 24
neurogenesis, 20, 28
neurologic disorders, 174
neurological disease, vii, viii, 14, 75, 77, 79, 92, 105, 114, 123, 166
neurological disorder, 174
neuromodulator, 150, 159
neuron death, 173
neuronal death, 168, 169
neuronal excitability, 135, 144
neuronal plasticity, ix, x, 125, 126, 139, 147
neurophysiology, 23
neuroprotection, 14, 79, 88, 92, 172
neuroprotective, 162
neuroscience, 93, 96
neurotoxic, 151, 161
neurotoxic effect, 161
neurotoxicity, 24, 79, 172
neurotransmission, viii, 39, 75, 78, 80, 81, 82, 92, 143, 150
neurotransmitter, 2, 4, 25, 76, 79, 80, 81, 92, 96, 103, 112, 137, 138, 154, 159, 165
neurotransmitters, ix, 26, 101
neurotrophic factors, 35, 76, 105
New England, 99
nickel, 156
nicotine, 49, 62, 68, 69, 73, 106, 115, 119, 123, 132
nigrostriatal, 109, 118
nitric oxide, 79, 86
NMDA, 127, 129, 131, 132, 133, 134, 135, 137, 141, 143, 146, 150, 156, 160, 162, 163, 170
NMDA receptors, ix, 9, 34, 56, 58, 70, 101, 108, 112, 116, 123, 127, 129, 131, 156, 160, 162, 163, 170
N-methyl-D-aspartate, 127, 142, 150, 172
N-Methyl-D-Asparte (NMDA), ix, 101
N-methyl-D-aspartic acid, 65
NMR, 85
nonsense mutation, 84, 85

Index

O

observations, 137
observed behavior, 103, 108
occlusion, 132
OH, 43
olfactory, 170
oligomers, 25, 32, 34, 119
open-field, 167
operations, 158
opioid, 132, 142
opportunities, 119
organ, vii, 1
osmolarity of fluids, vii, 1
overtraining, 111
oxidative stress, 77, 79, 87, 88, 92

P

PA, 171, 173, 174
pairing, 122
parallel, 123, 133
parenchyma, 151, 152, 153
parkinsonism, 25, 33
participants, 110
pathogenesis, 22, 23, 24, 105
pathology, 23, 24, 93, 112, 115, 122, 123
pathophysiology, 122
pathways, vii, 7, 9, 34, 62, 77, 78, 79, 90, 92, 102, 126, 127
PE, 144, 171
peptide, 21, 83, 98, 105, 119, 138, 151, 169
peptides, 23, 97
performance, 137, 175
perfusion, 7, 13, 21, 154, 161, 165
permeability, 8, 10, 17, 28, 169
permission, iv, 47, 48, 50, 51, 53, 56, 57, 58, 59, 60, 63
permit, 10, 60
peroxide, 88
personal, 126
personal relations, 126
personal relationship, 126
personality, 106
PF, 172
PG, 175
pH, vii, 1
phagocytosis, 24
pharmacological, 132
pharmacological treatment, 3
pharmacology, 47, 64, 95, 142, 146
phenomenology, 122
phenotype, 120
phosphatases, 129
phospholipase C, 160
phosphorylation, viii, 11, 15, 21, 27, 43, 45, 55, 58, 59, 62, 63, 64, 69, 70, 80, 87, 88
physiological, 158, 168
Physiological, 61, 175
physiological correlates, 109
physiological mechanisms, 25, 103, 106
physiology, 92, 95, 96, 167, 173
PI3K, 11, 13, 15, 27, 31, 82, 84, 88, 89, 91, 92, 96
pituitary, 164, 173
plants, 150
plasma, 151, 152, 165, 169, 175
plasma membrane, 4, 9, 34, 49, 88, 96, 151
plasma proteins, 151
platform, 83
play, x, 133, 137, 149, 160
plexus, 151, 152
PM, 99
polar, 4
polymerization, 88
pools, 85
population, 3, 109, 111, 165
pore, 127
positive correlation, 47
positive feedback, 138

norepinephrine, 136
normal, 151
novelty, 164, 174
nucleus, 34, 49, 67, 72, 81, 88, 107, 126, 128, 139, 140, 141, 142, 143, 144, 145, 146, 147, 153
null, 137, 158
nutrition, 174

187

188 Index

PTEN, 79, 87, 92
psychostimulants, 49, 138
psychosis, 145
psychology, 145
psychological stress, 164, 165, 173
psychoactive drug, 132
psychoactive, 132
psychiatric disorders, 80
PSD, 136, 140, 141, 146, 147
Prozac, 132
proteolysis, 87
proteins, ix, 8, 9, 21, 22, 25, 26, 33, 73, 76, 77, 78, 79, 80, 87, 94, 95, 97, 99, 151, 167
protein-protein interactions, 87
protein synthesis, 7, 15, 20, 39, 47, 83, 88
protein kinases, 13, 66, 127
protein kinase C, 21, 30
protein, 127, 129, 130, 135, 136, 142, 144, 151, 152, 169, 172
protection, 82
proteasome, 22, 23, 28, 30, 32
prostaglandins, 26
promoter, ix, 89, 102
project, 128, 130
pro-inflammatory, 26
prognosis, 106
probe, 110
probability, 2, 79, 80, 81, 85, 91, 113
primate, 93, 122
prevention, 25, 166
presynaptic, x, 149, 150, 156, 158, 159, 162, 163, 168, 170, 171
press, 170
preparation, iv, 46, 145, 153
pregnancy, 165
prefrontal cortex, 68, 93, 94, 126, 138, 141, 142, 143, 144, 145, 146, 147
preference, 132, 133, 142, 144, 145, 146
prediction, 133
preclinical, 147
PPI, 128
potassium, 20, 26, 135, 141, 159, 172
postsynaptic, x, 149, 151, 154, 156, 159, 160, 162, 163, 164, 168

Q

quality of life, 115
quinolinic acid, 107
Quinones, 144

R

RA, 169, 171
rain, 151, 152, 154, 167
range, 151, 154
rat, 140, 141, 143, 144, 145, 146, 147, 151, 152, 154, 155, 158, 159, 167, 168, 169, 170, 171, 172, 174, 175
rats, 138, 140, 142, 144, 146, 151, 152, 153, 164, 165, 167, 168, 169, 172, 173, 174, 175
RB, 170
RC, 171, 175
RE, 66, 67
reactive oxygen, 87
reactivity, 173
reagents, 2, 9, 157
reality, 123
receptor agonist, 136, 172
recognition, 81, 84, 85, 86, 95, 98
recommendations, iv
recovery, 53, 77, 90, 121
rectification, 10, 17, 18
recycling, 6, 21, 158
redistribution, 28, 38, 146
reduction, 135, 136
regenerate, 76
regeneration, 35, 81, 88, 89, 90, 91, 115, 118
regional, 161, 162, 167
regulation, 128, 171, 175
reinforcement, 128, 137, 142
reinforcement learning, 137, 142
relationships, 126

Index

S

SA, 171, 173, 174
saturation, 3
scaffolding, 136
scaling, 2, 3, 7, 12, 13, 14, 16, 18, 19, 20, 21, 22, 23, 24, 27, 30, 31, 32, 37, 38, 39, 40, 132
schizophrenia, ix, 76, 79, 80, 84, 97, 98
sclerosis, x, 149, 166
SE, 142, 174
secretion, 23
sedative, 71
seizure, 23, 27, 36, 166, 173, 174
seizures, 164, 165, 173, 174
selectivity, 52, 123
sensing, viii, 33, 75, 76, 78, 80, 86, 96
sensitivity, 95, 136, 139, 142, 175
sensitization, 66, 72, 73, 133, 134, 137, 140, 142, 143, 145, 146, 147
sensor proteins, 93, 95, 98
sensors, 8, 22
series, ix, x, 125, 131, 134
serotonin, 142
serum, 166, 167, 175
services, iv
sex, 126
SH, 168
sham, 90
shape, 47, 76, 77, 79
shares, 136
short-term memory, 119
showing, 92
signal transduction, 99
signaling, 127, 128, 143, 159, 163, 171
signaling pathway, viii, 4, 7, 8, 12, 14, 34, 44, 45, 76, 77, 78, 79, 81, 90, 92, 99, 127, 159
signaling pathways, 127
signaling, 30, 40, 94, 119
signals, 16, 78, 118, 153, 155, 156, 157, 163
signs, 109
silver, 150, 167
siRNA, 19
Slovakia, 98
smooth muscle, 69
smooth muscle cells, 69
social problems, ix, x, 125
sodium, 2, 5, 10, 17, 127, 132, 135, 147, 154
somata, 47, 93
SP, 169, 172
spatial, 127, 147, 158, 161, 172
spatial learning, 83, 147, 158
spatial memory, 28, 47, 66, 67, 81, 83, 96
species, 23, 25, 87

relevance, 118
relief, 115
remodelling, 94
repair, 82
reparation, 145
reperfusion, 170
repetitions, 112
replication, 167
repression, 35
researchers, 14, 23, 92, 165
residues, 8, 22
respiration, vii, 1
respiration rates, vii, 1
response, vii, 1, 5, 6, 12, 13, 18, 22, 23, 24, 26, 51, 52, 55, 60, 68, 72, 80, 81, 83, 84, 85, 86, 90, 92, 103, 104, 112, 114, 133, 139, 141, 144, 153, 154, 162, 164
responsiveness, 131, 138, 145, 165, 173
retardation, 84, 85, 96, 166
reticulum, 78
returns, 132
rewards, vii, 1, 126
RF, 145
rhythm, 67, 173
rights, iv
risk, 109, 121
risk factors, 109
RL, 142
RNA, 10, 17, 20, 33, 35, 37, 85
rodents, 83
root, 91
routes, 172
rules, 72, 95

189

Index

spectroscopy, 85
speech, 109, 121
spinal cord, 67, 89, 90, 94, 105, 110
spine, 16, 30, 36, 37, 38, 76, 77, 78, 79, 86, 93, 95, 103, 146
spleen, 89
sprouting, 84, 88, 89, 90, 91
SS, 69, 171
stability, vii, 1, 4, 7, 12, 37, 79, 137
stabilization, 103
standard error, 56
state, 19, 23, 37, 46, 51, 112, 113, 126, 132
states, 27, 139
stimulant, 147
stimulation, 9, 47, 53, 79, 80, 81, 90, 102, 103, 104, 107, 108, 110, 111, 112, 114, 115, 116, 117, 119, 120, 122, 123, 131, 140, 151, 155, 156, 157, 158, 159, 160, 162, 163, 164, 168, 170, 173
stimulus, viii, 43, 47, 53, 60, 81, 104, 131
storage, 79, 140, 167
strength, 127, 128, 131, 134, 135, 136, 137, 138, 140, 141, 144
stress, 77, 88, 92, 104, 118, 132, 134, 141, 144, 145, 146, 147, 164, 166, 173, 174, 175
stress response, 164, 173
striatum, 79, 104, 106, 107, 109, 111, 118, 122, 136, 137, 141, 144, 170
stroke, x, 149, 166
structure, 9, 66, 85, 95, 105, 144
subcortical nuclei, 104
substantia nigra, 170
substrate, 3, 55, 132
substrates, 72, 88
Sun, 32, 147, 172
supply, 152, 166
suppression, 5, 7, 16, 17, 18, 19, 28, 39, 159, 163
surface area, 76
survival, 31, 79, 87, 88, 92, 94, 123
susceptibility, 36, 166
swelling, 172
symptoms, viii, 25, 44, 46, 49, 61, 62, 92, 107, 109, 111, 115, 120

T

tangles, 24
target, 22, 38, 62, 71, 83, 85, 95, 129, 130, 134
tau, 24, 27, 99
technical assistance, 64
techniques, 7, 13, 53, 135
technologies, 115
temperature, vii, 1
temporal, x, 149, 164, 166
temporal lobe, x, 149, 164, 166
temporal lobe epilepsy, x, 149, 164, 166
terminals, x, 29, 92, 96, 137, 149, 153, 155, 156, 158, 159, 168, 170
testing, 122
tetanus, 136
TF, 172
thalamus, 105
theory, 147
therapeutic approaches, 115
therapeutic benefits, 97
therapeutics, 118
theta, 173

Index

thoughts, 103
time, 133, 154
tissue, 93, 104, 131, 168, 169
TJ, 143, 144
TM, 141, 146
TNF, 24, 26, 32, 36, 39
TNF-alpha, 36, 39
TNF-α, 24, 26
tones, 138
tonic, 39, 44, 80
topology, 8
toxic, x, 149, 161, 163
toxic effect, 52
toxicity, 52, 156, 162
toxin, 108
trace elements, 174
trafficking, 5, 6, 8, 9, 11, 13, 15, 16, 17, 19, 21, 25, 27, 28, 29, 30, 32, 33, 34, 35, 36, 37, 38, 39, 41, 50, 66, 72, 82, 86, 96, 98, 130, 136, 143, 144
training, 123
traits, 36, 111
trans, 172
transcript, 130
transcription, 14, 20, 25, 26, 41, 142, 167
transcription factor, 142, 167
transcription factors, 167
transfection, 81
transfer, 152
transferrin, 151
transition, 152
translation, 20, 31, 35, 36, 38
translocation, 13, 91, 96, 151, 158, 162, 164, 168, 170
transmission, vii, ix, 9, 25, 72, 75, 78, 84, 103, 106, 107, 110, 127, 132, 133, 134, 137, 138, 140, 141, 142, 145, 146, 168, 171, 174
transport, 24, 25, 26, 31, 49, 88, 151, 152, 154, 169, 170
treatment, 3, 7, 13, 15, 17, 19, 20, 23, 45, 48, 49, 52, 54, 61, 68, 69, 71, 73, 85, 88, 92, 99, 106, 107, 110, 131, 132, 138, 145, 147, 173
tremor, 109

triggers, 2, 11, 18, 24, 31, 113, 132, 158, 160
tumor, 31, 34, 39
tumor necrosis factor, 31, 34, 39
turnover, 11, 22, 34, 150, 154

U

ubiquitin, 22, 25, 30, 31, 32
ubiquitin-proteasome system, 22, 30, 31
uniform, 83
United States, 36, 105
universality, 94
USA, 1, 32, 39, 43, 65, 68, 99, 101, 117, 125, 171
UV, 169

V

vagus, 88
vagus nerve, 88
variables, 115, 131
vascular dementia, 39
vector, 89
versatility, 94
vertebrates, 103
vesicle, 4, 9, 80, 81, 158
vesicles, 150, 154, 158, 171
visuospatial function, 109
vitamin A, 28
vulnerability, 37, 123, 172

W

walking, 109, 121
Washington, 125
water, 44, 83
weight loss, 25, 166
white blood cells, 85
wild type, 85, 87, 88, 107
withdrawal, viii, 43, 44, 45, 46, 48, 49, 52, 54, 55, 56, 57, 60, 61, 62, 63, 64, 65, 68, 70, 71, 72, 73, 87, 88, 133, 135, 142, 145, 147

191

Index

withdrawal symptoms, viii, 43, 61, 62
working memory, 84, 118, 138
worms, 83

Z

Zinc, x, 149, 150, 151, 152, 153, 154, 155,
156, 158, 159, 160, 162, 164, 165, 166,
167, 168, 169, 170, 171, 172, 173, 174,
175
Zn, 168, 169, 170

zinc, vii, x, 149, 150, 151, 152, 153, 154,
155, 156, 157, 158, 159, 160, 162, 163,
164, 165, 166, 167, 168, 169, 170, 171,
172, 173, 174, 175